GLOBAL MENTAL HEALTH

RUTGERS GLOBAL HEALTH
Series Editor: Javier I. Escobar

GLOBAL MENTAL HEALTH

Latin America and Spanish-Speaking Populations

EDITED BY

JAVIER I. ESCOBAR, MD

RUTGERS UNIVERSITY PRESS

New Brunswick, Camden, and Newark, New Jersey, and London

Library of Congress Cataloging-in-Publication Data

Names: Escóbar, Javier, editor.
Title: Global mental health: Latin America and Spanish-speaking
     populations / edited by Javier I. Escobar.
Description: New Brunswick: Rutgers University Press, [2020] |
     Series: Rutgers Global Health | Includes bibliographical references and index.
Identifiers: LCCN 2019012940 | ISBN 9781978810044 (hardback: alk. paper) |
     ISBN 9780813595917 (pbk.: alk. paper)
Subjects: LCSH: Mental health services. | World health. |
     Hispanic Americans—Mental health.
Classification: LCC RA790.5 .E78 2020 | DDC 362.196/89008968073—dc23
LC record available at https://lccn.loc.gov/2019012940

A British Cataloging-in-Publication record for this book is available from
the British Library.

∞ The paper used in this publication meets the requirements of the American
National Standard for Information Sciences—Permanence of Paper
for Printed Library Materials, ANSI Z39.48-1992.

www.rutgersuniversitypress.org

Manufactured in the United States of America

To my wife, children, and grandchildren.
With appreciation to the many dear colleagues who
have enriched the field of global mental health.

CONTENTS

SERIES FOREWORD

JAVIER I. ESCOBAR

This is the second volume from the series on global health published by Rutgers University Press. The focus on mental disorders reflects the relevance of these disorders globally in terms of their huge cost and the high level of disability that they induce. Unfortunately, global investment made in this area lags significantly below that made in other areas of health, such as infectious and nonmental diseases. The expansion of the field of global mental health during the last decade has been stimulated by small investments from foundations as well as a few research grants from the National Institutes of Health (NIH). These investments have resulted in fruitful collaborations, such as the global mental health "hubs" funded by the National Institute of Mental Health (NIMH) that were primarily focused on developing "task-shifting" strategies for helping with the shortage of specialty mental health professionals in low- and middle-income countries (LMICs). Very few of these global mental health collaborations have taken place in Latin America and the Spanish-speaking world.

The essays included in this volume represent a number of research collaborations in which the senior editor of this series (JIE) has engaged for the past two decades.

Besides providing a snapshot of the field of global mental health, the book highlights an important new model for assessing and managing mental disorders from a cultural perspective, and also presents some preliminary findings from exciting new collaborative research projects focusing on chronic, severe mental disorders in Latin America. This research is state-of-the-art and includes the training of new investigators in those regions, as well as sophisticated clinical and neurological assessments making use of leading technologies such as neuroimaging and genetic studies. The book also provides the recent history and caveats related to the abuse of psychiatry globally, with a particular emphasis on the occurrence of these abuses and misuses of psychiatry in Spanish-speaking countries.

GLOBAL MENTAL HEALTH

INTRODUCTION

The field of global mental health (GMH) is still quite young. Following the laborious anthropological and epidemiological work from many pioneers, the field has significantly expanded, particularly during the last decade. A growing number of recent books and publications focusing specifically on the topic of GMH attest to the maturing of the field.

Equity in services and support for the mentally ill, and capacity building, particularly in economically deprived regions of the world, have been guiding principles of the field in efforts to lessen disparities, particularly those affecting low- and middle-income countries (LMICs). A growing number of institutions, including governmental and nongovernmental organizations, have become actively engaged in these global initiatives. This has resulted in many fruitful collaborations and key developments, such as the "task-shifting" strategy leading to the implementation of evidence-based approaches to deal with mental health problems worldwide.

Most GMH collaborations in LMICs have taken place in African and Asian countries, with very few reports coming from Latin America and the Spanish-speaking world. Moreover, the focus of the work has been primarily on the services and capacity-building fronts, in efforts to attain equity and implement evidence-based approaches broadly. There has also been a clear emphasis on recognizing and managing mental disorders, taking advantage of the universally available primary care platforms and, in the process, engaging a broad a range of primary care workers in efforts to counter the existing deficits in numbers of trained mental health professionals in many regions of the world.

This book focuses primarily on a few selected examples from Latin America and the Spanish-speaking world. The selection of authors and essays for this book was based on direct experiences and collaborations of the book editor (JIE) with many investigators and colleagues at a number of global sites in the United States, Latin America, and Spain. The book, therefore, presents selected vignettes that target a handful of global initiatives in which the main editor has participated either directly or indirectly, rather than a comprehensive perspective of the field of GMH. These examples, however, provide interesting leads on a number of evidence-based interventions, the forging of true international collaborations, and the possibility of doing state-of-the-art research beyond equity and service concerns, as well as the potential for abuse of unrestrained mental health policies and interventions.

Chapter 1, "A Brief Review of Global Mental Health," is an introductory essay providing a panoramic review of the GMH field. It is authored by Stanley Nkemjika, MD, MPH, a physician specializing in public health and a postdoctoral fellow in global health; Javier I. Escobar, MD, MSc, the main editor of the book, an academic psychiatrist and global health administrator and researcher; and Humberto Marin, MD, a professor of psychiatry and a practicing clinician. All three authors are on the faculty at Rutgers–Robert Wood Johnson Medical School (RWJMS). This first chapter tracks the history and emergence of GMH and highlights challenges, critical issues, and major developments in the field. It also provides brief descriptions of metrics, diagnostic issues, and key interventions needed in GMH. Finally, it introduces the relevant topic of evidence-based interventions and their scope, promises, and limitations.

Chapter 2, "Looking at Cultural Aspects of Global Mental Health," is by Miwa Yasui, PhD, a clinical psychologist and an associate professor at the University of Chicago; and Kathleen Pottick, PhD, a social psychologist and social worker and a professor at Rutgers, The State University of New Jersey. The Culturally Infused Engagement model developed by Yasui, Pottick, and Chen is a globally relevant and innovative new model originally devised to practically guide cultural engagement and assessments for helping immigrants and people from various ethnic minorities in the United States. Intuitively, this model should have significant relevance for GMH interventions in many world populations. In this chapter, Yasui and Pottick provide a scholarly review of relevant cultural issues for Hispanic and Asian individuals in the United States and other countries that will serve as an important cultural frame for engaging and assessing diverse populations globally, with a particular focus on Latin American and Asian-origin populations.

Chapter 3, "The Abuse of Psychiatry Globally" by Ethan Pearlstein, a medical student at Rutgers-RWJMS, and Javier I. Escobar, MD, MSc, reviews the abuse of psychiatry from a historical and a global perspective. Besides the relevant and classic examples of the abuse of psychiatry in Nazi Germany and the Soviet Union, the review also highlights events in other countries, including Latin America and Spain. A major focus of the chapter centers on a highly relevant but little-known historical example of the abuse of psychiatry in Francoist Spain during and after the civil war in that country, a historical piece that the authors have been examining with interest in the last couple of years.

Chapter 4, "Task-Shifting Strategies in Latin America," is by Maria Calvo, MD, and Eduardo Padilla, MD, both psychiatrists from the mental health division in the region of Jujuy in Argentina; Mariana Figueredo Aguiar, an officer at the Fundación de Lucha contra los Trastornos Neurológicos y Psiquiátricos en Minorías in Buenos Aires, Argentina (FULTRA); Javier I. Escobar, MD, MSc; and Gabriel de Erausquin, MD, PhD, an Argentine-born psychiatrist who is professor and chair of neurology and psychiatry at the University of Texas, Rio Grande Valley. This chapter describes a successful U.S.–Latin American collaboration that has led to important research initiatives and the training of new local researchers to address mental health problems in the Andean region of Argentina. This research focuses on a special population of Quechua origin located high in the Andes Mountains near the border between Argentina and Bolivia. The chapter provides information on a highly effective "task-shifting" strategy imbedded in primary care and leading to an improvement in the early recognition and management of psychoses in the region. A consortium of investigators from Argentina, Peru, Bolivia, the United States, and the United Kingdom have collaborated in this endeavor.

Chapter 5, "Genetic Research on Chronic, Severe Mental Disorders in the Paisa Population in Latin America," is by Carrie E. Bearden, PhD, a professor and leading researcher from the Semel Neuroscience Research Institute at UCLA; Carlos Lopez Jaramillo, MD, professor and chair of psychiatry at the Universidad de Antioquia in Medellin, Colombia; and Javier I. Escobar, MD, MSc,. This chapter describes the "Paisa" population in Latin America and reports on a fertile collaboration of U.S. and Latin American institutions to study major mental disorders focusing on this special population. This collaboration has led to important research on Alzheimer's disease, bipolar disorder, and other major psychiatric disorders. The current NIH-funded research now taking place in Colombia and mentioned in this chapter focuses on eliciting genetic and endophenotypic characterization of severe mental disorders on that special population.

The final chapter, "A Brief Rejoinder and Future Directions," by Javier I. Escobar, MD, MSc, includes a brief agenda for future activities on behalf of global health in Latin America and the Spanish-speaking world.

1 · A BRIEF REVIEW OF GLOBAL MENTAL HEALTH

Challenges, Developments, and Needs

STANLEY NKEMJIKA, JAVIER I. ESCOBAR, AND HUMBERTO MARIN

BACKGROUND

Millennium Development Goals: The recent impetus of a global approach to health; followed the United Nations initiative on health objectives for the new millennium; launched in the year 2000.[1] These goals included:

- End of hunger
- Universal education
- Gender equity
- Child health
- Maternal health
- Combatting HIV/AIDS
- Environmental sustainability
- Global partnership

While it seems rather remarkable that problems related to mental health were not originally listed among these top priorities, in 2005 the World Health

Organization's European ministerial conference added the necessary sentence to correct this omission by stating, "There is no health without mental health."[2]

In 2009 a committee of the Institute of Medicine of the United States strongly endorsed the new millennium initiatives and recommended large investments to fulfill the Millennium Development Goals. Additional investments were also recommended to combat injuries and noncommunicable conditions such as heart disease.

Today, almost two decades after the goals were drafted, it must be acknowledged that even though some of the objectives have been at least partially fulfilled in many countries (e.g., ending hunger, improving universal education, improving child and maternal health, and combatting HIV/AIDS), severe problems and disparities continue to exist, particularly in low-income countries, and many of these problems currently occur on the mental health front.

Global Health: George Bernard Shaw's old dictum "There is no such thing as perfect health; nobody is ever really well" continues to resonate, despite countless efforts to define and catalogue the concept of health. The World Health Organization (WHO) defined health as "a state of complete physical, mental, and social well-being and not merely the absence of disease or infirmity," a broad, rather unrealistic definition that has not been modified since 1948. The concept of "health equity" and the attainment of the Millennium Development Goals have been central tenets to the notion of global health. As an area for study, research, and practice, global health places a high priority on improving health and achieving equity in health for all people worldwide. The Institute of Medicine has briefly defined global health as "health problems or concerns transcending national boundaries which may be influenced by circumstances or experiences in other countries and are best addressed by cooperative actions and solutions." The emphasis on cooperation across borders is, in our view, the essential ingredient in this definition.

Thanks largely to unprecedented opportunities such as the emergence of new donors and philanthropists, efforts could be initiated to promote excellence and equity in health-care delivery for poor, underserved populations globally. More specifically, a number of successful programs geared toward reducing morbidity and mortality from infectious diseases have been rejuvenated through the use of viable platforms that incorporate provisions to comprehensive health care for those exposed to poverty and chronic disease.[3]

Global Health and the U.S. Government: The U.S. government took a significant interest in global health in the past two decades, in particular during President Barak Obama's first term. Obama wisely stated, "The US global health investment is an important component of the national security smart power strategy" and even proposed a cabinet position in his administration to address health issues globally. Unfortunately, this initiative could not be realized due to political and budgetary issues, but it had a clear impact on a number of institutional settings, including academic medicine.

Global Health at the National Institutes of Health (NIH): Shortly following his appointment as NIH director in the early 2000s, Francis Collins, the scientist who led the project that catalogued the human genome, listed global health as one of his top four priorities for the organization and advocated the expansion of research efforts to aid developing nations and increasing research collaborations with low- and middle-income countries (LMICs). In early interviews following his appointment, Collins expressed a strong commitment to alter the view most countries had about the United States "by emphasizing the US role as that of a doctor rather than a soldier." Unfortunately, political and budgetary issues also brought this initiative to a halt. On the positive side, however, some global mental health initiatives and investments continued to be seen at various NIH institutes, particularly the National Institute of Mental Health (NIMH) and the NIH-Fogarty Institute, the international arm of NIH. Thus, some NIH institutes (NIMH among them) have facilitated global research by allowing RO1 grants, the prototypic and most-valued awards at NIH, to be carried out in foreign lands, thus making the RO1 granting mechanism a bit more accessible to international projects.

GLOBAL MENTAL HEALTH

The WHO defines mental health as "a state of well-being in which the individual realizes his or her own abilities, can cope with the normal stresses of life, can work productively and fruitfully, and is able to make a contribution to his or her community." The state of mental well-being includes cognitive, emotional, and attitudinal components. It is a continuum rather than a state that is either present or absent. Three components of mental well-being— emotional, psychological, and social—have been proposed. Definitions of mental health need to consider the attributes of each particular society, its needs, resources, social ideals, and values. Being mentally healthy refers primarily to the absence of mental distress or disease, specifically, the absence of a specifiable or diagnosable mental disorder.[4,5]

As many of these global mental health concepts and constructs have evolved from values endorsed by Western Europeans and North Americans, beyond literal translation, they need to be properly adjusted and calibrated before they are applied to other world regions and countries. Certain psychological and behavioral components appear to be universal, however, such as the "positive" traits of altruism, respect, and ability to relate to others or to consider the needs of others. Also, "negative" traits such as violence, lack of regard for others, and antisocial behavior are universally discouraged. Moreover, severe mental disorders such as mania and psychoses appear to be clearly differentiated and recognized in most cultures.

Critical Issues for Global Mental Health

Currently, the most pressing mental health issues globally include:

- Early identification of disorders and interventions for those in need
- Access to quality mental health care for all
- Integration of mental health and primary care services
- Scientific collaborations

—Early identification of mental disorders is critical and carries prognostic value. As availability of mental health professionals is scarce in many regions, primary care workers need to be properly trained, and individuals with mental disorders should be helped to recognize and understand their illnesses through such processes as psychoeducation. This empowerment lessens stigma and helps those suffering from mental disorders to pursue available therapeutic options and to access information on the effectiveness and side effects of potential treatments, ideally, as part of a process of shared decision making.[6]

—Regarding access to services, the mental health needs of a population should be ideally fulfilled in an equitable, accessible, and acceptable manner. Building on the advances of research on the management of mental disorders, the promotion and strengthening of a wide network of support resources that are evidence-based and geared toward recovery and prevention are essential.[7,8] These approaches attempt to address and correct the enormous health disparities and disadvantages that exist in many regions of the world regarding the provision and quality of mental health care, and they reinforce respect for the human rights of people with mental disorders globally.[9,10]

—A significant improvement in delivering mental health services can be achieved through integrating mental health care into existent primary care programs, yet true integration is lacking in most countries, including the United States. For most vulnerable groups, such as those plagued with intellectual disabilities and those with chronic and severe mental disorders such as schizophrenia and dementia, there is an urgent need for more research, for adequate resources toward the provision of acute care management, for cost-effective and continuous follow-up strategies, and community resources to aid deinstitutionalization of those with chronic mental health problems. A more coherent and cordial interaction between specialists and nonspecialists is needed for these efforts to reach their true potential. This integration may revolutionize the care of the mentally ill through facilitating clinical care and management and reducing global inequalities to health care access.[7,8]

—To achieve a balance between high-income and low-income countries, the field also needs to address transnational influences on mental health such as migration, conflicts, disasters, and the impact of global trade policies. Although much remains to be achieved, the successful proliferation and implementation of global health projects in selective low- and middle-income nations should serve as a pilot and a model for mental health care delivery in other regions as forecasted by the Movement for Global Mental Health.[11]

Global Burden of Mental Disorders

What follows are critical and challenging statistics pointing to the heavy burden that mental disorders impose globally.

—Mental illness constitutes an estimated 7.4 percent of the world's measurable burden of disease.[12]

—The economic burden of mental disorders exceeds those of the four major categories of noncommunicable diseases: diabetes, cardiovascular diseases, chronic respiratory diseases, and cancer.[13]

—Major depression is the second-leading cause of years lived with disability (YLDs).[14]

—Anxiety disorders, alcohol/drug disorders, schizophrenia, and bipolar disorder rank among the twenty medical conditions contributing the largest global share of YLDs.[14]

—The human resource gap exceeds one million mental health workers in LMICs.[10]

Prevalence of Mental Disorders Globally: At the start of the new century, it was estimated that, on average, one out of four people worldwide would experience a mental health or neurological anomaly at some point in their lives.[15] Starting in the 1990s, mental disorders have been increasingly recognized as one of the leading sources of disease burden and disability in communities around the world. More recent epidemiological studies, such as the world mental health surveys, confirm the high overall prevalence of mental disorders.[16] Indeed, a single mental disorder, depression (as a broad syndrome), is the second-most common cause of disability worldwide, after back pain (a rather ambiguous and heterogeneous medical condition). The cost and level of disability induced by severe mental disorders is very high and is dependent upon early age of onset, as many of the chronic, severe mental disorders such as schizophrenia start during adolescence or early adulthood, hence hampering individuals' ability to function efficiently during their most productive years. Concurrently, there is considerable evidence that environmental contingencies such as poverty, exposure to violence, social exclusion, or inequalities are all key social determinants of mental illness, thus placing disadvantaged individuals at much greater risk for mental disorders.[17]

WHO Metrics and the Global Burden of Disease (GBD): Measuring disease and injury burden in populations requires a composite metric that captures premature mortality, the prevalence and severity of ill health, and the degree of functional impairment and disability. In 1990, the WHO launched the Global Burden of Disease (GBD) project, which proposed the disability-adjusted life years (DALYs) measure to assess disease burden globally. DALYs incorporate the sum of years of life lost (YLLs) and years lived with disability (YLDs). While the term *disability* has taken on many meanings in different settings of the GBD lexicon, it is generally used to catalogue any short-term or long-term health loss other than death. The concept of "health" in the GBD context is defined in terms of overall functioning, which encompasses multiple health domains such as mobility, pain, affect, and cognition. Quantifying health loss in terms of DALYs has led to placing increased attention on mental health problems, particularly once major depressive disorder began moving up in the health rankings, on its way to becoming one of the top health problems globally by the first decade of the twenty-first century. The WHO reported that mental disorders represent more than 13 percent of the global burden of disease, surpassing both cardiovascular disease and cancer. Specifically, depression was noted to be the third-leading contributor to the global burden of disease currently, and it is projected to be second overall by 2025; alcohol and illicit drug use account for more than 5 percent of the global burden as well. These statistics depict the huge impact that mental disorders have on the global burden of disease. Among the reasons for this unique impact of mental disorders on global burden, we should mention the early onset and lifetime course of many of these disorders, the limited knowledge of their pathophysiology and therapeutics due to incomplete understanding of the brain and its mechanisms (both molecular and cellular), and the absence of successful preventive interventions.

A BRIEF OUTLINE OF KEY GLOBAL HEALTH AND GLOBAL MENTAL HEALTH INITIATIVES

Partners in Health (PIH) is a laudatory example of a nongovernmental organization (NGO) that has shown remarkable success in the achievement of millennium goals. The PIH's amazing growth from the early 1980s to the present was generated by the collaboration, over time, of physician-anthropologists Paul Farmer and Jim Yong Kim (who was president of the World Bank). The foundational framework, as detailed in several publications, was primarily ethnographic and anthropological.[18] PIH initially focused on Haiti, and after becoming a "super" NGO globally is now aimed at scaling up effective delivery systems worldwide. PIH's initial projects took place in Cange, Haiti, and other marginalized regions of the world. By working in these low-income, resource-poor regions, Farmer and collaborators quickly realized that the traditional approach to health did not apply in those places and that it was imperative to develop innovative approaches that would consider culture, geopolitical structure, and the overwhelming relationship connecting poverty to health in order to properly understand health problems and implement solutions globally. Without incorporating such considerations, Farmer and colleagues concluded, it would not be feasible to offer quality health care or address the many existing challenges to global health in many world regions. PIH has become a pioneer in successfully recognizing and managing a number of the most stubborn afflictions of underserved communities throughout the world, such as HIV/AIDS, tuberculosis, cancer, and other ailments. PIH has opened new paths for effective, high-quality health care through collaboration with governments and communities and the formation of health worker networks, a process that has been implemented even in communities in need within the United States. One outstanding example of the impact of the PIH approach has been the African country of Rwanda, a country that within one decade has achieved the most dramatic gains in population health and poverty reduction in the world, including the full realization of the health-related Millennium Development Goals. According to Farmer and his foundation, "These outcomes serve as a beacon, exemplifying what can result when visionary leaders relentlessly pursue evidence-based care through robust health systems, with particular emphasis in rural populations" (Paul Farmer, personal communication). One happy end product of this effort in Rwanda has been the development and construction of a novel global university, the University of Global Health Equity.

Grand Challenges in Global Mental Health Initiative: In efforts to address the severe problems faced by many LMICs, the Grand Challenges in Global Mental Health initiative was launched by a consortium of international agencies including the U.S. National Institute of Mental Health (NIMH) in Bethesda, Maryland, and the Global Alliance for Chronic Diseases (GACD), headquartered in London. This consortium identified research priorities for the ensuing decade that were thought to have an important role in improving the lives of people living with mental disorders. A key goal of these interventions was that they should have a global scope. This initiative was one of the first to utilize the Delphi method, a structured technique using controlled feedback in efforts to arrive at consensus using a dispersed panel of participants. Other major objectives were to cover the full range of mental disorders and eventually build a wide-ranging community of research funders and researchers.

In an important paper published in the journal *Nature*, [19] Pamela Collins, then deputy NIMH director, together with several collaborators from across the world, outlined these challenges and proposed some solutions:

- Identify root causes, risks, and protective factors for mental disorders
- Advance prevention and implementation of early interventions

- Improve treatments and expand access to care
- Raise awareness of the global burden
- Build human resource capacity
- Transform health systems and policy responses[19]

Thanks to this initiative, NIMH's international research, which had been traditionally restricted to HIV research during the 1980s to 2000s, expanded to other fronts. Thus, in the mid-2000s, NIMH started funding "collaborative hubs" in Africa, Asia, and Latin America. NIMH also launched other global initiatives, such as "RFA-MH-16-350," that were intended to foster research partnerships for scaling mental health research in LMICs.

The main emphasis of the NIMH research investment was on integrating mental health into primary care platforms, making resources more readily available to mental patients in those countries, and placing an emphasis on "equity in access to, quality of and outcomes of mental health care worldwide."[19]

Also, some initiatives at the NIH-Fogarty institute, such as "Brain Disorders in the Developing World: Research across the Life Span" and "Mobile Health Technology in Low- and Middle-Income Countries," did significantly contribute, among other things, to the training of a new cadre of researchers in LMICs.

The *Lancet* Initiative on Mental Health: The *Lancet*, a leading international medical journal, launched a series of articles on the topic of GMH focused on building upon the levels of evidence outlined above. Vikram Patel, an India-born psychiatrist who practiced in the United Kingdom, led this movement. The excerpts from the *Lancet* series on GMH have been adopted as a focus of action toward the field of GMH and have led to highly visible initiatives such as the WHO's Mental Health Global Action Program (mhGAP) and the Movement for Global Mental Health.[20-22]

The Mental Health Resource Gap: Over 80 percent of the global population resides in LMICs and has access to less than 20 percent of the share of the mental health resources available globally. Similarly, resources for mental health research are also limited, and knowledge gaps still persist, as well as shortfalls in trained mental health professionals; these deficits are the backdrop to an unprecedented treatment gap for mental disorders in low-income countries, with over 75 percent of patients left untreated. This huge gap in mental health access and service availability affects the most basic human rights, as more than 75 percent of individuals in LMICs suffering from major anxiety, mood disorders, or substance-use disorders receive suboptimal or no care at all, despite their significant functional disability. Sub-Saharan Africa alone has a huge treatment gap for schizophrenia and other psychotic disorders that exceeds the 90 percent mark, due to lack of services as well as substandard access to the few existing services.[23] A major problem related to mental health in many areas of the world, particularly in LMICs, is the scarcity of specialized mental health professionals such as psychiatrists, psychologists, psychiatric nurses, or psychiatric social workers. This tremendous gap is also currently seen in highly developed countries such as the United States. Evidence-based approaches in many countries must be anchored in primary care. This includes the proper training and supervision of primary care practitioners (physicians, nurses) or even primary care workers (trained community members) so that they can help recognize and manage common mental disorders. This "task-shifting" strategy will be discussed in detail later in this chapter. One of the key goals of these new initiatives in capacity building is the early recognition and effective management of major disorders including psychotic disorders such as schizophrenia as well as severe mood disorders.

The WHO's mhGAP initiative was primarily geared toward scaling up services for people with mental, neurological, and substance-use disorders in many countries, particularly those with low- and middle-income levels. It proposed that despite the scarce resources that exist in many areas, major mental disorders could be managed with properly trained personnel, leading to the provision of psychosocial assistance and medications. The mhGAP program is designed to promote an evidence-based platform to train nonspecialist health workers to recognize and properly manage eight mental, neurological, and substance-use disorders in routine health care settings.[23]

Movement for Global Mental Health: This has been defined as "a network of individuals and organizations that aim to improve services for people living with mental health problems and psychosocial disabilities worldwide, especially in low- and middle-income countries where effective services are often scarce."[22] Two key principles are scientific evidence and human rights.

The Movement for Global Mental Health is a worldwide coalition of individuals and institutions committed to implement actions that mitigate and improve the treatment gap. Awareness on mental disorders and their consequences has been on the rise, as institutions, governmental bodies, and private donors have pledged endowments to the field. Through active collaborations with other health disciplines, the members of the Movement for Global Mental Health coalition have contributed significantly to the promotion of personal and communal well-being, the prevention of mental illness, and the provision of effective, ecologically sustainable mental health interventions for those in need around the world.[22]

Other Unique Global Mental Health Initiatives: It is also helpful to highlight the launching of several other academic initiatives globally, such as those from the Center for Global Mental Health in London.[24] Also, there have been important capacity-building initiatives in global mental health led by academic institutions such as the master's program in international mental health policy, services, and research at the University of Lisbon, in Portugal; and in the United States, the already mentioned Grand Challenges in Global Mental Health initiative led by the National Institute for Mental Health and the Global Alliance for Chronic Diseases.[19]

Despite the above developments, there is still plenty of room for expanding GMH, as investments in this area remain quite small, despite the overwhelming need, compared to other areas of health such as infectious or cardiovascular disease. Big donors such as the Gates Foundation have been, in general, quite reticent to invest in the area of GMH, possibly because of the complexity and the subjective nature of psychiatric diagnoses and the absence of reliable and measurable markers to assess outcomes.

Global Mental Health Research: Regarding GMH research, there has been little progress in truly understanding the etiology, pathophysiology, and treatment for most mental disorders from a global perspective. According to the experts, future breakthroughs will depend on new discoveries in genomics and neuroscience. While by necessity GMH research initially focused on disease-burden reduction, impact on equity, immediacy of impact, and feasibility of interventions, there has to be an effort to embrace new developments in the neurosciences. The information gathered thus far from "services research" particularly focused on capacity building should serve as a focal point for immediate research and prioritization of policies, as incremental progress in addressing the grand challenges in GMH should bring significant economic and quality-of-life benefits.

THE ROAD TOWARD A MATURE FIELD OF
GLOBAL MENTAL HEALTH

Culture and Global Mental Health: Human beings are immersed in environments where they acquire the ability to function and co-exist, first as children, then most importantly as adults, through a series of developmental processes that are heavily controlled and influenced by forces operating within the culture. Culture is part of the essential fabric of health, and it plays an essential role in shaping individual perceptions, structural inequalities, distribution of resources, and other issues that may lead to health disparities, as well as the adoption of negative attitudes toward mental disease, such as stigma and discrimination. Culture is also pivotal to symptom formation and interpretation, and it has a powerful impact in shaping the form, course, and outcome of mental disorders. It is also a key determinant for the doctor-patient relationship, an essential dyad influencing the acceptance of medical advice and the adherence to prescribed medical interventions.

Within a given community, culture includes local and global elements transmitted via local and transnational networks. It may be true that many cultural differences are fading through the role of globalization, increased mobility of populations, telecommunications, and globalized economic forces. However, the impact of globalization appears to be too complex for many people to grasp effectively. This has resulted in an increase of cultural hybridization and a broad range of cultural variation within single societies and countries. Cultural elements impacting GMH appear to be closely related to overriding economic and social factors that cause poverty, discrimination, inequality, and adversity. Hence, many mental health problems may have their roots in sociodevelopmental processes, difficult interactions with others, or deleterious environments.

Culture shapes all illness experiences and influences ways in which distress or discomfort is expressed and communicated across different cultures. Thus, every culture has its own health repertoire, manifested in the form of unique "idioms of distress," which are culturally sanctioned modes of expressing personal suffering that are intelligible and comprehensible to others within the same community.[25,26] Knowledge about nonmedical ancillary local systems of healing is also essential for understanding the logic of local patterns of help seeking, pathways that people follow to care, as well as the goals, benefits and potential problems associated with specific treatment methods.[27]

While it is vital to be aware of local values and norms, the naïve devaluation or overvaluation of local or "indigenous" GMH practitioners and interventions is problematic. The recognition of the cultural complexity of ethical issues within the broad context of global inequality makes a further demand on those engaged in GMH to be increasingly flexible and skeptical as they assess and re-examine their own practices and contrast them with other views of the world.

A great majority of existing mental health problems and issues, including psychoses, mania, depression, anxiety, addictions, somatic or dissociative symptoms, have been described globally, with broad arrays of explanations for the phenomena being exhibited across different cultures. Thus, in many cultures, laypeople view mental disorders as related to moral weakness, religious influences, personal challenges, or as the consequences of family or community discord.[28] These views may contribute to the stigma carried by many of these disorders.

Prognosis of severe mental disorders such as schizophrenia has been reported to vary globally. Previous research sponsored by the WHO such as the international pilot study of schizophrenia (IPSS)[29] documented different illness outcomes that were related to specific world regions. The better or more optimistic prognosis for schizophrenia seen in developing societies was originally attributed to the presence of more communal, less individualistic approaches, and possibly to a more tolerant, less demanding attitude toward the mentally ill. Unfortunately, no new research of this type has been implemented in the decades since the results of IPSS were published. The impact of economic development and globalization may be changing the outcome picture, as evidenced in a recent report from China by Chunping Ni and colleagues, based on a survey that collected data from more than two million people. According to this report, schizophrenia disability in China has almost doubled in two decades, and it is affecting rural populations more than urban populations, thus reversing previous trends, possibly reflecting the deep changes undergone by Chinese society in recent decades.[30]

Anthropology and Global Mental Health: Historically, an important perspective in global mental health has been the anthropological approach. This approach originally focused on the description of exotic syndromes from distant lands, advanced important theories concerning the "emic" (from phonemics, meaning local) and "etic" (from phonetics, meaning universal) perspectives on mental disorders. A number of true pioneers in this area must be mentioned here. This list includes several anthropologists and cultural psychiatrists in the United States, such as Arthur Kleinman, Byron Good, Janice Jenkins, and Marvin Karno.

Arthur Kleinman, an American physician and anthropologist at Harvard, has been a leading figure in medical anthropology and cultural psychiatry and also a pioneer for global mental health. He conducted research in China and in Taiwan from 1969 until 1978 and produced important reports on psychiatric disorders such as neurasthenia.

Byron Good, an anthropologist also at Harvard, was interested in examining how culture and social structure impact the course and the presentation of psychiatric disorders. Good had a special interest in Indonesia and has been involved in building and evaluating mental health services in this and other low-resource settings in Asia. He is a former editor in chief of *Culture, Medicine, and Psychiatry*, an important international journal on the field of medical anthropology.

Marvin Karno, a professor at UCLA, was one of the pioneers of Hispanic mental health in the United States. He has mentored many global scholars throughout the years, including the editor of this book. Karno also led the Los Angeles Epidemiologic Catchment Area Project, a pivotal NIH-funded survey examining Hispanic and non-Hispanic populations. He has always shown particular interest in immigrants from Mexico and Latin America. He opened the first clinic in the United States serving Mexican immigrants.[31]

Janice Jenkins, an anthropologist who worked with Marvin Karno at UCLA, has also done important work on global cultural aspects of mental disorders such as schizophrenia in Latin American patients. She is also the editor of an authoritative textbook on the topic of global mental health.[32]

A recent book, *Global Mental Health: Anthropological Perspectives*, provides an updated view of the promises and intricacies of the anthropological approach, in efforts to dispel perceptions such as the one suggesting that the traditional "emic" approach may be "patronizing," as a majority of the leading "emic" investigators have come from Westernized countries.[33] Indeed, the passionate focus of some investigators from high-income countries (such as the United States) in combating stigma and helping to build up, improve, or integrate mental health services in LMICs abroad, while commendable, often ignores the fact that in their own country the availability and integration of mental health and primary care services are still quite deficient. It is not therefore surprising that Paul Farmer and his PIH have also focused their hands-on approach to work on deprived areas of the United States, as part of programs aimed at addressing health problems in impoverished and neglected areas of the country, such as the PIH/COPE program in the Navajo nation of the Southwest and the PIH/PACT program near Boston.

Going from the "Exotic" to the Mainstream: In today's globalized world, following massive waves of migration and the assemblage of giant communication networks, there is a clear turnaround from the local to the universal. Thus, many of the formerly "unique" syndromes described by anthropologists and cultural psychiatrists have become more permeable and have lost their well-defined boundaries, as they are being increasingly seen and recognized in many countries and cultures, even in those that are highly developed. The "etic" or universal approach gained special impetus following studies sponsored by the WHO showing that major psychiatric disorders can be reliably identified in most countries and cultures and that psychiatric resources such as the American Psychiatric Association's *Diagnostic and Statistical Manual of Mental Disorders* (DSM-5) and, particularly, the International Classification of Diseases (ICD) appear to have universal acceptance and appeal. The fact that the "emic" perspective may be losing ground does not alter the obvious impact that cultural background still has on the presentation, treatment preferences, and treatment response of mental disorders across the globe.

Relevant Publications on Global Mental Health: In the recent past, there have been several other relevant publications in the area of global mental, a majority of them coming from England. This list includes:

—*Global Mental Health: Principles and Practice,* edited by Vikram Patel, an India-born psychiatrist practicing in England, and a group of collaborators.[34]
—*The Palgrave Handbook of Sociocultural Perspectives on Global Mental Health,* also from England.[35]
—"Anthropology and Psychiatry: A Contemporary Convergence for Global Mental Health," a chapter in the second edition of the *Textbook of Cultural Psychiatry,* edited by Dinesh Bhugra and Kamaldeep Bhui, in the United Kingdom.[36]

In the United States, two publications that should be noted are:

—*Essentials of Global Mental Health,* edited by Samuel O. Opakpu in 2014 and *21st Century Global Mental Health,* edited by Elliot Sorel in 2016.[37,38]

The appearance of many of these publications—together with the global mental health research investment of NIH, the WHO, NGOs, and other organizations—represents the coming of age for global mental health. These developments have corrected, among other things, the original perception that mental disorders were a Western idealization, and they have documented the painful realities that these disorders bring all over the world and the global burden resulting from them. Moreover, a few innovative evidence-based interventions such as "task-shifting" strategies embedded in primary care, first tried in low-income countries, appear to work well universally. This should facilitate the recognition and management of mental disorders with state-of-the-art pharmacological and psychotherapeutic approaches.

Implementation Approaches

Implementation Research and Implementation Science (IS): Implementation research is extremely relevant to global health because it addresses the challenges of the existing gap in services worldwide and the practical achievement of national and global health goals. This approach involves the creation and application of knowledge to improve the implementation of health policies, programs, and practices using multiple disciplines and methods. It emphasizes key partnerships between the implementation team, community members, researchers, and policy makers. It involves practical approaches to facilitate implementation of initiatives to enhance equity, efficiency, buildup, and sustainability, with the ultimate goal of improving people's health.[39,40]

In GMH, implementation science (IS) contains the knowledge base needed to optimally embed and sustain effective mental health interventions within clinical and community systems. These include training of health care workers, integration of mental health into primary health care, improving the access and the supply of effective medications and redesign of health care systems. These components are all badly needed to overcome both supply and demand barriers to evidence-based care.[40]

The emergence of coordinated GMH research efforts across a range of institutions (WHO, NIMH, Canadian Development Agency, and others) can be credited for these initiatives, and leaders at the WHO and the World Bank now rely on IS for many other initiatives. While some projects have already succeeded in embedding services within LMICs, additional strategies are still needed to scale up these efforts across the grassroots. This synergy of GMH and IS activities creates an ideal platform to form an implementation network that will advance the knowledge base through:

—Identifying key outcomes by researchers and practitioners
—Applying existing IS frameworks to LMIC contexts
—Identifying common data elements and core components of effective interventions, as well as tools for researchers and practitioners to identify key questions
—Establishing collaborative multisite studies such as those exemplified by the five-country PRIME project on integrating mental health into primary care in LMICs and the various NIH-funded collaborative projects or "hubs" in Africa, Asia, and Latin America.

One "hub" reaching significant visibility in the field was the South Asian Hub for Advocacy, Research, and Education on Mental Health (SHARE).[41]

Also, NIH-funded hubs of particular relevance to Latin America are the LATIN MH Network[42] and the Regional Network for Mental Health Research in Latin America, RedeAmerica. It is unclear whether or not these hubs are still functional and what the outcomes of such interventions in countries such as Argentina, Brazil, Chile, and Colombia have been.

As part of these major efforts for meeting basic mental health needs globally, there is growing interest in embedding evidence-based mental health interventions within alternative delivery structures such as schools and primary care systems and the delivery of mental health services by community health workers and other paraprofessionals, particularly in LMICs.

Information Technologies: An exciting innovation is that brought about by mental health information technologies through the use of tablet and PDA-based assessments. This has made it possible to quickly and effectively screen for mental disorders, and it also facilitates the delivery of several interventions via audiovisual devices (smartphones) such as individual counseling and structured psychotherapies.

Telepsychiatry: More recently, telepsychiatry is also making an importance entrance, both locally and globally, and it seems that this field will continue to grow exponentially. Moreover, this may also facilitate long-distance training and supervision of lay workers. While these advances show great promise, they will have to be properly tested and evaluated to examine their impact on health outcomes globally.

SPECIAL ISSUES IN GLOBAL MENTAL HEALTH

Global Mental Health and Immigration: Migrants, displaced populations, and refugees are all common worldwide. In the United States, traditionally a country of immigrants, research on the mental health consequences of migration has led to disparate findings. Initially, immigration research started with pivotal papers by O. Odegaard and others in the 1940s to the 1950s.[43,44] Odegaard's reports were based on the study of hospitalized patients in the then-burgeoning state hospital system in the United States. These and other publications from those early years suggested that immigrants were at a much higher risk for mental disorders compared to the U.S.-born population.[45,46]

Two decades later, however, research focusing on Mexican immigrants showed totally different results. William Vega and other investigators in California showed that Mexican immigrants to the United States had lower rates of major mental disorders, particularly alcohol- and substance-use problems, than their U.S.-born counterparts.[47] Research reports on other health areas besides mental health, as well as mortality statistics, also documented the fact that despite significant disadvantages and disparities, Latino immigrant groups fared significantly better than the U.S.-born, leading to the formulation of the "Latino paradox."[48]

Interestingly, in the United Kingdom (UK), immigration has been traditionally associated with poor mental health, and a number of studies on patients hospitalized with severe mental disorders (psychosis) also showed an excess of psychosis among immigrants, particularly those from Jamaica.[49-54] It is suspected that the excessive diagnosis of psychosis in the UK may be related to diagnostic bias, similar to what has been observed in the case of African American patients in the United States.[55]

Information on the mental health consequences of immigration in other European countries shows that Turkish immigrants in Germany were reported to present a higher frequency of mental disorders such as anxiety and personality disorders, psychosomatic disturbances, and abnormal psychological reactions compared to the general population.[56] In Spain, psychiatric symptoms in immigrants have been largely attributed to discrimination.[57] However, a more recent study of immigrants and native Spaniards in the Aragon region of Spain showed that the Spanish-born had a higher overall prevalence of mental disorders, particularly substance-use disorders compared to the immigrant groups.[58]

Translation in Global Mental Health: Translation of texts, documents, and procedures is an important process in GMH. The merits of translation are highlighted in the preface of the first English edition of the King James Version of the Bible, possibly the most translated instrument in the history of mankind, which includes the following passage: "Translation it is that openeth the window, to let in the light; that breaketh the shell, that we may eat the kernel; that putteth aside the curtain, that we may look into the most holy place." However, it must be acknowledged that translation is a complex process. A sentence found in the legendary novel *Don Quixote* states that "translating from one language to another is like looking at Flemish tapestries from the wrong side, for although the figures are visible, they are covered by treads that obscure them and cannot be seen with the smoothness and the color of the right side." Many years ago, as part of epidemiological research, the senior author of this chapter (JIE) learned firsthand the nuances and complexities of the translation process when he participated in the translation, adaptation, and community use of a psychiatric diagnostic instrument, the Diagnostic Interview Schedule (DIS), that was used in a national study of psychiatric disorders in the 1980s. The state-of-the-art methodology for translation and adaptation of instruments was articulated by Richard W. Brislin in the 1970s, a process that needs to consider cultural, conceptual, and structural equivalence plus the use of back translation as well as review by cultural and linguistic experts. Regarding language and translation issues, anthropologists have raised the issue of "working understandings," perhaps a convenient way to avoid the rigors of literal and conceptual translations. This approach contends that despite the shortfalls of perfect, fully accurate translation, assurance of full equivalency and proper adaptation across cultures and languages, it may be possible to devise efficient ways of working that can limit or allow for the correction of errors in order to meet the specific requirements of clinical or research contexts. The senior author has highlighted many of the issues that impact the translation of psychiatric classifications and criteria (DSM-5) in a recent publication.[59]

Psychiatric Classifications: DSM-5 and the International Classification
of Diseases (ICD)

A critical need globally is to have standardized systems for assessing and clas-
sifying mental disorders. Two key international instruments are the fifth
edition of the *Diagnostic and Statistical Manual of Mental Disorders* (DSM-5),
the official psychiatric nomenclature in North America,[60] and the International Classification of Diseases (ICD) of the World Health Organization
(WHO) developed for global use.[61]

DSM-5: The fifth revision of the DSM system appeared in 2013. DSM-5,
the official psychiatric diagnostic instrument in the United States, is also utilized across the world particularly for research purposes. DSM-5 had significant input from international experts. To American psychiatrists, ICD is of
utmost current importance, as ICD-10 is the official system for coding and
billing purposes in the United States. Fortunately, the DSM-5 developers took
this into account and in the fifth revision, each DSM-5 diagnosis has corresponding ICD-9 and ICD-10 CM codes. The fact that the ICD-10 codes are
already in DSM-5 facilitated the task of shifting from ICD-9 to ICD-10. However, this does not necessarily mean that there is a perfect diagnostic corre-
spondence between DSM-5 and ICD-10.

DSM-5 Cultural Formulation: This initiative has been led by Roberto
Lewis Fernandez, a psychiatrist at Columbia University, and it is included
in the DSM-5, providing guidelines for assessing and managing patients from
different cultural and ethnic backgrounds.[61]

ICD-11: The WHO is currently developing the eleventh edition of the
international classification (ICD-11). It is expected that given the international input and interest in DSM-5 and the ongoing consultation between
APA and the WHO, the final version of ICD-11 will resemble the DSM-5 to
a larger degree than the ICD-10 classification resembled the DSM-IV. ICD-11
is currently under development and has not yet been officially released. It
originates and expands from a set of basic points and agreements between
mental health professionals.[62]

Similarly to what was also the goal with DSM-5, new technological
advances should help keep ICD-11 as a "living document," experiencing
transformations when new significant information coming from different
environments and stakeholders arrives rather than a complete, periodic,
rewriting of the criteria, as has been the tradition until now. Due to the

scarcity of data coming from "best available science" that could be used to inform psychiatric classifications, utility, reliability, and some equivalents to validity will be the core guiding principles of ICD-11. The ICD-11 approach intends to convey a considerable amount of clinically relevant information about the disorder, including both essential and typical features, differential diagnosis, the boundary with normality, typical course, and developmental and cultural-specific features.

A procedure called "prototype matching" consists of clinicians estimating to what extent the patient's clinical presentation matches a paragraph-length description of the disorder; this concept will be utilized for ICD-11.

The proposed categories or blocks for ICD-11 are the following: neuro-developmental disorders, schizophrenia and other primary psychotic disorders, catatonia, mood disorders, anxiety and fear-related disorders, obsessive-compulsive and related disorders, disorders specifically associated with stress, dissociative disorders, bodily distress disorder, feeding and eating disorders, elimination disorders, disorders due to substance use, impulse control disorders, disruptive behavior and dissocial disorders, personality disorders, paraphilia disorders, factitious disorders, neurocognitive disorders, psychological and behavioral factors affecting disorders or diseases classified elsewhere, mental and behavioral disorders associated with disorders or diseases classified elsewhere, sleep-wake disorders and symptoms, and findings and clinical forms of mental and behavioral disorders.

DSM-ICD Harmonization: One of the most sensitive issues about this harmonization project is whether ICD should resemble DSM or DSM resemble ICD. Perhaps in some instances the harmonization should go in one direction (e.g., DSM to ICD, while in others it may go in the opposite direction (ICD to DSM). The necessary comparison between both systems and the decision that one would prevail over the other creates competition and adds sensitivity to the process. No matter how logical these DSM-ICD relationships sound, problems and debates will continue to arise among proponents or detractors of either system. Clearly these matters cannot be resolved using only empirical data, and at the end, harmonization may become a political issue. Although harmonization between ICD-11 and DSM-5 is one of the main goals articulated by the developers and potential users of each of these systems, it is likely that significant differences across the two systems will remain at the end. However, it is hoped that these differences will not be as remarkable as those reported for ICD-10 and DSM-IV.[63-65]

DSM-5 in Spanish-Speaking Countries: While used primarily for the purpose of research, the new diagnostic system appears to work well in Latin American and Spanish-speaking countries. For example, a field trial of the new personality disorders category in the DSM-5, coauthored by the editor of this book (JIE), showed that the DSM-5 alternate classification for personality disorders, one of the most complex areas to assess in psychopathology, worked admirably well in the Basque-speaking population, a special population isolate in northern Spain.[66]

GLOBAL ASPECTS OF EVIDENCE-BASED PSYCHIATRIC PRACTICE

Evidence-Based Medicine (EBM): Nowadays the term EBM is used to designate a relatively recent approach to medical practice. The original concept arose on both sides of the Atlantic more than two decades ago. In the words of Sackett and colleagues, who wrote one of the pioneering papers on EBM, "Evidence-based medicine is the conscientious, explicit and judicious use of current best evidence in making decisions about the care of individual patients." They added that "by best available external clinical evidence we mean clinically relevant research . . . especially from patient centered clinical research."[67] EBM refers to the systematic application of the scientific method to basic and clinical research for the production of medical knowledge. This strategy, which started after the Second World War, has been led largely by the United States and thus is essentially an American creation. Although other countries now increasingly produce medical evidence, the United States continues to be its principal producer and exporter, and the model used to produce scientific evidence is basically the American model. Evidence-based approaches include both proof of efficacy and estimation of the risks of the interventions.

As stated in a recent perspective written in the *New England Journal of Medicine*, "Physicians still drew on their own experiences and instincts, but evidence-based medicine enabled them to expand their personal proof models with broader data sets and less bias."[68]

While it is undeniable that this initiative has had a very positive and significant impact on medical practice and in the transmission of medical knowledge, it should be emphasized that the concept, when used narrowly, applies mainly to the treatment of individual patients in medical practice. Moreover, the concept has been constantly evolving since the field went from intuitive medicine to evidence-based medicine. In fact, a recent publication is already proposing "personalized medicine" as the next step beyond EBM.[68]

The modern scientific method of medical research seems now so obvious and natural to most of us that even those versed in the history of medicine have problems accepting the reality that the systematic enforcement of evidence in medical practice started only by the middle of the twentieth century, 250 years after the invention of the steam engine, 60 years after the production of the first car, and almost simultaneously with the production of the first atomic bomb.

Federal monitoring of medical treatments formally began in October 1962, when the U.S. Congress passed the Kefauver Harris amendment to strengthen drug regulation, including demonstrating efficacy, reporting adverse effects, and establishing consent from participating subjects. In an ideal world, all drugs, all devices, and all medical treatment techniques that are prescribed to patients should demonstrate evidence of being both effective and safe.

However, this is far from being fully accomplished yet, due at least in part to the following:

• A large fraction of current medical practice is not based on evidence, a problem more dramatic in specialties such as psychiatry and other mental health disciplines.
• A substantial number of preparations, devices, and techniques used with therapeutic purposes remain exempt from premarketing safety and efficacy standards such as those that are now mandatory for new drugs.
• There exist variable, often questionable standards to determine efficacy, as well as different standards to determine "efficacy" and "effectiveness," with little or very loose application of the essential concept of "contextual efficacy."
• It remains difficult to adjudicate the truthfulness and relevance of many evidence-based approaches, due to conflict of interest and other sources of bias.

Food Supplements and Folk Remedies: From a societal point of view, one of the most problematic issues in the health and mental health areas is the indiscriminate use of food supplements and folk remedies, such as herbs. This is due to the high number of people using these substances, including many children, and the lack of formal approval or supervision for their use. In fact, calling them "food supplements," as the law permits in the United States, sounds like a cruel irony, because in the United States at least, supplements are less regulated than food. From a global perspective, add to this the complexities of translation of a plant's name or genus, especially from countries that have non-Roman alphabets, such as China and other Asian countries. The next hurdles are related to the lack of formal or official controls during production, contamination of supplements with bacteria or chemical compounds, especially insecticides, and the fact that in the case of some supplements, such as Ayurvedic medicines, contamination with heavy metals may be intentional.

Definition of Efficacy: Surrogate Standards of Efficacy and Application of the Concept of Contextual Efficacy

Medical treatments are primarily intended to prolong life, improve function, and increase quality of life. However, in clinical studies, surrogate or proxy measurements of efficacy are the ones most commonly utilized—for example, the requirement to reach a certain number or threshold to determine efficacy on a metric scale for assessing clinical effects of psychiatric or pain medications. A frequent point of uncertainty in this regard is where exactly to set the numeric threshold. While statistical tests are applied to decide whether an intervention is effective or not, in many cases, the magnitude of change in a particular scale required to demonstrate statistical efficacy may not yield major practical gains if it doesn't correlate with significant improvement in real-life conditions. Thus, many interventions may be statistically but not practically "significant." A potential solution to this problem is the use of real-life endpoints such as life prolongation, functional status (days worked, days hospitalized), and quality of life. However, because this latter strategy is more difficult and costlier to implement, it is often not included in many trials.

The concept of contextual efficacy is a reminder that interventions, such as drugs or psychotherapy, are not used in a vacuum but with real patients, living in a specific time, in particular living conditions, and usually with access to alternative therapeutic options. Therefore, judgments on the efficacy and risks of interventions need to consider the concomitant use of other agents (pharmacological, nonpharmacological) to which individuals are often exposed simultaneously with the new intervention.

There are several other issues that may interfere with scientific discourse and the establishment of evidence-based approaches locally and globally:

—Denaturalizing medical evidence through plain falsification, adulteration, distortion, or adoption of commercial terminology, instead of standard scientific definitions. This often takes the form of manipulation of the evidence, with "cherry picking" of the results or the silencing or attenuation of negative findings.

—Conflict of interest. The means by which scientific discourse is conducted have been unduly influenced by the interests of multiple constituencies. These include journals without proper peer review, particularly those whose main purpose is to profit from revenues coming from authors, their institutions, or pharmaceutical companies, which may lend a veneer of science to otherwise meaningless results.

Large-Scale Treatment Studies: Results from pivotal studies funded by NIH such as CATIE, STAR-D, and others have shown no major differences between very costly new drugs (such as the many atypical antipsychotics) and older, less expensive ones (antipsychotics such as fluoperazine or haloperidol) in terms of efficacy, effectiveness, effects on cognition, quality of life, or discontinuation rates.

Unfortunately, in the United States, federal funds such as those coming from the National Institute of Mental Health (NIMH) to support services research, including large-scale research projects as those mentioned above, have been drying up. Moreover, the political will of official entities to make forceful decisions that impact medical practice seems to be fading with the rise of a deregulation movement that sees as "toxic" any governmental opinion or intervention that interferes with the "free" action of economic forces.

Possible Silver Lining: The National Center for Advancing Translational Sciences (NCATS), a new development at the National Institutes of Health (NIH), was recently established to catalyze a transformation in the way health interventions are developed and to bring more treatments to more patients more efficiently and quickly. This includes a large network of more than fifty academic medical centers (hubs). With the goal to expedite clinical trial processes from start-up to close-out, NCATS has established the NCATS Trial Innovation Network (TIN). The TIN is a collaboration that joins three Trial Innovation Centers (TICs), a Recruitment Innovation Center (RIC), and the Clinical and Translational Science Award (CTSA) program hubs. The goal of the TIN is to conduct high-quality multisite clinical trials faster and more cost-efficiently through the provision of services such as institutional review boards (IRB) and standard contract agreements or by helping investigators develop robust recruitment and retention plans. In addition, the TIN serves as a national laboratory to study, understand, and innovate the process of conducting clinical trials and to accelerate the translation of novel interventions into life-saving therapies. We certainly hope that these developments at NIH can be sustained and expanded, to the benefit of evidence-based medicine and psychiatry.

EVIDENCE-BASED PSYCHIATRIC APPROACHES FOR GLOBAL USE

General Issues for Applying Evidence-Based Interventions Globally

As previously described, epidemiological research has documented the enormous burden related to mental disorders globally, with major depression, schizophrenia, bipolar disorder, and substance-use disorders being among the top ten contributors to years lived with disability. It is thus imperative to focus on the recognition and proper management of these severe, chronic disorders worldwide.

The growth of well-documented evidence-based practices—including the efficacy and effectiveness of several pharmacological and well-defined and monitored psychological approaches for managing chronic, severe mental disorders, coupled with the effective training and development of nonspecialist health care workers who could deliver evidence-based psychological interventions for mental disorders—has offered attainable global solutions for recognizing and managing mental disorders in regions lacking sufficient resources. However, implementation of needed programs and interventions has been a difficult and tortuous process. Thus, traditional interventions such as Freudian psychoanalysis, which was created in the late nineteenth century and became the predominant therapeutic instrument at least in the United States until the late 1960s, continue to be practiced and taught worldwide, despite very limited evidence-based support. Even worse, several other so-called psychotherapies currently in use today have either a poor evidence base or no scientific base at all. Some of these, such as "recovery memory therapy" and "conversion therapy" (the latter, a largely discredited effort to change the sexual orientation of gay people) have led to unfortunate medical and social tragedies. Thus, many current practices in the field of mental health are not based or anchored in evidence, and this includes not only psychotherapeutic but also pharmacological approaches.

Task-Shifting: The key concept of task-shifting has had a monumental role in shaping global mental health interventions worldwide. The results of most of these projects have demonstrated that mental health care can be delivered effectively in primary health-care settings through community-based programs using task-shifting approaches. "Task-shifting" is the name given to a process of professional delegation whereby specific tasks are reassigned to lower-level, less-specialized health workers. This process may also entail employment of mental health care providers in primary care sectors and collaborations with non–health care professionals in order to strengthen mental health awareness, detection of mental disorders, proper implementation of referrals, and effective service delivery. Task-shifting represents a useful, practical approach that can be used by public health agencies and national governments to address the issue of shortages of trained professionals especially in LMICs. A key paper that appeared in the *Lancet* in 2011 illustrated the gap that exists between high- and low-income countries and the dramatic need worldwide for trained mental health professionals.[10] According to this publication, while nurses represent the largest workforce category in the mental health system, followed by psychiatrists and psychologists, their numbers are remarkably low in many regions of the world. The numbers of social workers and occupational therapists are also alarmingly low. Psychiatrists are far more prevalent in high-income countries as compared to low-income countries. Through reorganizing the workforce and adding community workers, task-shifting presents a viable solution for improving health care coverage irrespective of a country's economic power by making more efficient use of the human resources already available in communities and by quickly increasing capacity while training and retention of specialized professionals are expanded.[7]

Psychotherapeutic Approaches Globally: An article published in 2013 in *Public Library of Science* (PloS) *Medicine* and editorialized in *Nature*, a leading scientific journal, identified seven specific subtypes of psychotherapy that appeared to meet evidence-based standards globally.[69,70] These are interpersonal psychotherapy (IPT), cognitive-behavioral therapy (CBT), behavioral-activation therapy (ACT), problem-solving therapy (PST), psychodynamic therapy (DYN; a brief intervention different from traditional psychoanalysis), social skills training (SST), and supportive counseling (SUP). All seven were found to yield better results than control conditions.

Myrna Weissman, a professor at Columbia University, is an authority on psychiatric epidemiology and one of the developers of IPT. She has coauthored an authoritative textbook on the topic.[71] Weissman has also contributed to the global front in an important collaboration with the WHO.[72] Interestingly, in a recent paper published in the *American Journal of Psychiatry*, Weissman highlights the fact that the use of effective forms of psychotherapy is growing exponentially in many countries of the world while fading in the United States.[73] Thus, psychotherapy is becoming less accessible in the United States, despite the STAR-D project's demonstration that CBT was as effective as drug treatment as a second-step treatment for depression.

The use of psychotherapy in low-income countries has targeted primarily depression, the most prevalent GMH problem worldwide. Other important evidence-based global data highlighted by Weissman includes the following:

—ITP has been used for the treatment of depression in Uganda, a country seriously affected by HIV and civil war. The treatment's positive results in reducing depression and sustaining the effects could be widely disseminated.[74]

—A clinical trial was also successfully completed in Goa, India, using ITP to treat depression in primary care.[75]

—The Canadian government supported training of health workers in Ethiopia for administering ITP embedded in general health care, and still another Canadian grant helped scale up a stepped-care model for treatment of depression that includes brief psychotherapy embedded in the primary care network of Partners in Health, Paul Farmer's original initiative in Haiti.

—Another important evidence-based intervention was the clinical trial of CBT administered by community health workers in rural Pakistan that found a reduction in mothers' symptoms at six months in the CBT group, results that were sustained for up to one year.[76]

—A randomized, controlled, clinical trial of CBT for patients with repeated primary care consultations due to medically unexplained symptoms in general medical clinics in Sri Lanka found that CBT was feasible and effective in reducing symptoms of distress and number of visits.[77]

Managing Schizophrenia and Other Psychoses: The high cost of "atypical" antipsychotics has limited their broad global use, and therefore the "old" or "typical" neuroleptics remain as the ones most commonly prescribed in many countries of the world. Fortunately, the tradition in most LMICs has been the use of relatively low dosages of neuroleptics, in contrast to the high dosages of these agents originally employed in the United States. Among the effective interventions for psychoses that may be expanded globally, we wish to mention the use of long-acting neuroleptics for the proper maintenance of rigorously diagnosed and well-documented schizophrenic syndromes. Long-acting neuroleptics are among the most effective and yet one of the most underutilized interventions for managing schizophrenia worldwide, even in the United States.

Also, the addition of family management approaches has been documented to universally enhance the therapeutic potential for interventions on chronic, severe mental disorders such as schizophrenia or bipolar disorder.

Drug Treatment of Depression: In the case of depression, the judicious use of effective dosages of antidepressants can be coordinated through primary care systems worldwide. Indeed, even in the United States, most antidepressants are not prescribed by psychiatrists but by primary care physicians, and this is even more significant in LMICs. In general, the use of relatively low dosages of one of the specific serotonin receptor inhibitors (SSRIs) such as fluoxetine, citalopram, or sertraline is recommended as the first-line treatment for depression of at least moderate severity worldwide.

Evidence-Based Interventions: Focus on Latin America
and the Spanish-Speaking World

The total population of Latin American and Caribbean countries is now estimated to exceed 600 million people. If we include Spain, countries such as the United States where Spanish is spoken as a second language by more than 40 million people, and the twenty Latin American countries where Spanish is the official language, it is estimated that more than 500 million people speak Spanish, making it the third-most-spoken world language after English and Mandarin. As can be inferred from the above reports, with a few exceptions, little work on evidence-based interventions has had a specific focus on Spanish-speaking populations.

Renato Alarcon, a leading Latin American psychiatrist, reviewed the state of Latin American mental health more than a decade ago.[78] Regarding the mental health workforce, he reported that in the first decade of the twenty-first century, resources in Latin America were very limited, with average estimates of 1.7 psychiatrists, 2.7 psychiatric nurses, 2.8 psychologists, and 1.9 social workers per 100,000 people, numbers far below those reported from Europe or the United States. He also listed several urgent needs that existed in Latin America at that time, including support for training and research, integration of mental health and primary care services, increase in the mental health workforce, and support from international agencies and organizations.[78]

In Chile, Ricardo Araya, Graciela Rojas, and their team of investigators have produced important evidence-based research particularly focused on treatment of depression in primary care.[79] Also in Chile, a nationally mandated plan has promoted the integration of mental health into primary care clinics, an effort that appears to be successful at least in the short term.[80]

Two of the coauthors of this chapter (HM and JIE) wrote a paper several years ago on the psychopharmacological management of Hispanic American patients, and this included some recommendations and caveats for managing mental health problems in Latino populations both inside and outside the United States.[81] These included general instructions to practicing clinicians such as:

—Be kind, respectful, and formal. While respecting boundaries, become a friend. For many Latin American patients, trust is a most personal and relevant matter.
—Do not take for granted the empowerment and autonomy of the patient, and assess the degree of participation that makes him or her comfortable.
—Ask about food supplements and folk remedies. Latin Americans are huge utilizers of these.
—Keep in mind that Latin American patients generally have higher expectations about drug treatments and may respond better to them.
—Start at low dosages. Latin American patients may be more sensitive to psychiatric medications due to less previous exposure to them.

Besides listing the several recommendations and caveats for treatment approaches to Latin American patients, that paper also highlighted a pioneer comparative study in the United States and Colombia done by the senior editor of this book (JIE) in the 1980s. That study, comparing two antidepressants (imipramine and trazodone) to a placebo using a double-blind design, showed similar results in the two countries but suggested that at the dosages used, imipramine seemed to work better in the Colombian subjects compared to those in the United States.[82] South American patients appeared also to have more anticholinergic side effects to imipramine than the U.S. subjects. Observations during the same study also showed significant differences in symptom presentations of depression between North American and South American patients.[83]

GENERAL CONCLUSIONS

Mental illness is frequent, is costly, causes severe functional impairment, and significantly increases mortality worldwide. It is surrounded by stigma, and its management and outcome are clouded by the unfortunate perpetuation of the Cartesian dichotomy.

On the positive side, the United Nations has given a high priority to the attainment of key health indicators as part the 2015 Sustainable Development Goals (SDGs) and the WHO consensus of European Ministers has eloquently stated that "there is no health without mental health."

The WHO, NIH, Canadian Institutes, the World Bank, and private foundations (the Gates Foundation and others) have been investing in the global health field. Unfortunately, investments made on the global mental health front remain very small compared to those for other areas of health.

The task-shifting strategy and the community health workers initiatives that originally focused on low-income countries are now being successfully applied globally to deal with shortages of medical and mental health specialists. This model may be applicable even to countries such as the United States.

While effective, evidence-based interventions are available for some disorders, the outcomes of many interventions have not been thoroughly investigated or evaluated using the scientific method, and their efficacy and cost-effectiveness remain largely unknown.

Integration of care, an important priority, has not been universally embraced and remains quite tenuous, even in high-income countries such as the United States. The example from Chile presented earlier remains as a model for the continent, and we hope it can be expanded to other countries.

A final positive commentary: The significant increase in the number of scholars and students entering the field—full of youth, energy, and academic enthusiasm—that we have observed in the past decade augurs a bright future for the field of global mental health.

REFERENCE LIST

1. World Health Organization. Millennium Development Goals; 2000.
2. World Health Organization. *The European Health Report 2005: Public Health Action for Healthier Children and Populations.* Geneva: WHO; 2005.
3. Gilbert BJ, Patel V, Farmer PE, et al. Assessing development assistance for mental health in developing countries: 2007–2013. *PLoS Med.* 2015;12(6):e1001834.
4. Tucker DK, Harding le Richie W. Mental health: The search for a definition. *Can Med Assoc J.* 1964;90(20):1160–1166.
5. Manwell LA, Barbic SP, Roberts K, et al. What is mental health? Evidence towards a new definition from a mixed methods multidisciplinary international survey. *BMJ Open.* 2015;5:007-079.
6. Costello J. Early detection and prevention of mental health problems: Developmental epidemiology and systems of support. *J Clin Child Adolesc Psychol.*2016;45(6):710–717.
7. Patel V, Prince M. Global mental health: A new global health field comes of age. *JAMA.* 2010;303(19):1976–1977.
8. Thornicroft G, Deb T, Henderson C. Community mental health care worldwide: Current status and further developments. *World Psychiatry.* 2016;15:276–286.
9. World Health Organization. *Investing in Mental Health.* Geneva: WHO; 2003.
10. Kakuma R, Minas H, van Ginneken N, et al. Human resources for mental health care: current situation and strategies for action. *Lancet.* 2011;378:1654–1663.
11. Fiskin A, Miglani M, Buzza C. Implications of global mental health for addressing health disparities in high-income countries. *Psychiatric Annals.* 2018;48(3):149-153.
12. Murray C, Vos T, Lozano R, et al. Disability-adjusted life years (DALYs) for 291 diseases and injuries in 21 regions, 1990–2010: A systematic analysis for the global burden of disease study. *Lancet.* 2012;380(9859):2197–2223.
13. Bloom DE, Cafiero-Fonseca ET, Candeias V, et al. Economics of non-communicable diseases in India: The costs and returns on investment of interventions to promote healthy living and prevent, treat, and manage NCDs. World Economic Forum, Harvard School of Public Health; 2014.
14. Vos T, Flaxman AD, Naghavi M, et al. Years lived with disability (YLDs) for 1160 sequelae of 289 diseases and injuries 1990–2010: A systematic analysis for the Global Burden of Disease Study 2010. *Lancet.* 2012;380:2163–2196.

15. World Health Organization. The world health reports 2001: Mental health; new understanding, new hope. Geneva: WHO; 2001.

16. Steel Z, Marnane C, Iranpour C, et al. The global prevalence of common mental disorders: A systematic review and meta-analysis 1980–2013. *Int J Epidemiol.* 2014:43(2): 476–493.

17. Kessler RC, Berglund PA, Bruce ML, et al. The prevalence and correlates of untreated serious mental illness. *Health Service Research.* 2001;36:987–1007.

18. Farmer P, Kleinman A, Kim J, Basilico M, eds. *Reimagining Global Health: An Introduction.* Berkeley: University of California Press; 2013.

19. Collins PY, Patel V, Joestl SS, et al. Grand challenges in global mental health. *Nature.* 2011;475:27–30.

20. Global Health Burden 2013 Collaborators. Global, regional, and national incidence, prevalence, and years lived with disability for 301 chronic diseases and injuries in 188 countries 1990-2013: A systematic analysis for the Global Burden of Disease Study. *Lancet.* 2013;386:743–800.

21. World Health Organization. Mental Health Action Plan: 2013–2020. http://www .who.int/mental_health/publications/action_plan/en/www.who.int.

22. Movement for Global Mental Health website. http://www.globalmentalhealth.org.

23. World Health Organization. WHO Mental Health Gap Action Programme. http://www.who.int.mental.health.mhgap.

24. Center for Global Mental Health, London. http://www.centreforglobalmental health.org.

25. Lewis Fernandez R. Cultural formulation of psychiatric diagnosis. *Culture Medicine and Psychiatry.* 1996;20(2):133–144.

26. Karno M, Jenkins JH. Cross cultural issues in the course and treatment of schizophrenia. *Psychiatric Clinics of North America.* 1993;16(2):239–250.

27. Escobar JI. Transcultural aspects of dissociative and somatoform disorders. *Psychiatric Clinics of North America.* 1995;18:555–569.

28. Raviola G, Becker AE, and Farmer P. A global scope for global health—including mental health. *Lancet.* 2011;378:1613–1615.

29. Jablensky A, Sartorius N, Ernberg G, et al. *Schizophrenia: Manifestations, Incidence, and Course in Different Cultures: A World Health Organization Ten-Country Study.* Psychological Medicine Monograph Supplement 20. Cambridge: Cambridge University Press; 1992.

30. Ni C, Ma L, Wang B, Yan Y, et al. Neurotic disorders of general medical outpatients in Xian, China: knowledge, attitudes, and help-seeking preferences. *Psychiatr Serv.* 2014;65:1047–1053.

31. Karno M, Edgerton RB. Perception of mental illness in a Mexican-American community. *Arch Gen Psychiatry.* 1969;20(2):233–238. doi:10.1001/archpsyc.1969.01740140105013.

32. Jenkins JH. *Extraordinary Conditions: Culture and Experience in Mental Illness.* Berkeley: University of California Press; 2015.

33. Kohrt BA, Mendenhall E. *Global Mental Health: Anthropological Perspectives.* Walnut Creek, Calif.: Left Coast Press; 2015.

34. Patel V, Minas H, Cohen A, Prince M. *Global Mental Health: Principles and Practice.* New York: Oxford University Press; 2013.

35. White RG, Jain S, Orr DMR, Read U, eds. *The Palgrave Handbook of Sociocultural Perspectives on Global Mental Health.* London: Palgrave Macmillan; 2017.

36. Bhugra D, Bhui K, eds. Anthropology and psychiatry: A contemporary convergence for global mental health." In: *Textbook of Cultural Psychiatry.* 10th ed. Cambridge: Cambridge University Press; 2018.

37. Opakpu SO, ed. *Essentials of Global Mental Health.* Cambridge: Cambridge University Press; 2014.

38. Sorel E., ed. *21st Century Global Mental Health.* Burlington, MA: Jones & Bartlett Publishers; 2013.

39. Betancourt TS, Chambers DA. Optimizing an era of global mental health implementation science. *JAMA Psychiatry.* 2016;73(2):99–100.

40. Theobald S, Brander N, Gyapong M, et al. Implementation research: New imperatives and opportunities in global health. *Lancet.* 2018; October 9 https://doi.org/10.1016/S0140-6736(18)32205-0.

41. South Asian Hub for Advocacy Research and Education on Mental Health (SHARE). http://www.sharementalhealth.org.

42. Latin American Treatment and Innovation Network in Mental Health (LATINMH). National Institute of Mental Health. http://www.latinomh.com.br/.

43. Odegaard O. The incidence of mental disease as measured by census investigation versus admission statistics. *Psychiatric Quarterly.* 1952;26:212.

44. Odegaard O. *Emigration and Insanity.* Acta Psychiat. Neurol., Suppl. 4; 1932.

45. Dunham HW. *Community and Schizophrenia: An Epidemiological Analysis.* Detroit: Wayne State University Press; 1965.

46. Srole L, Langner TS, Michael ST, et al. *Mental Health in the Metropolis: The Midtown Manhattan Study.* New York: McGraw-Hill; 1962.

47. Vega WA, Kolody B, Aguilar-Gaxiola S, et al. Lifetime prevalence of DSM-III-R psychiatric disorders among urban and rural Mexican Americans in California. *Arch Gen Psychiatry.* 1998;55(9):771–778.

48. Escobar J, Hoyos-Nervi C, Gara M. Immigration and mental health: Mexican Americans in the United States. *Harvard Review of Psychiatry.* 2000;8(2):64–72.

49. Wessely S, Castle DJ, Der G, et al. Schizophrenia and Afro-Caribbeans: A case-control study. *Br. J. Psychiatry.* 1991;159:795–801.

50. Bhugra D, Leff J, Mallett R, et al. Incidence and outcome of schizophrenia in Whites, African Caribbeans, and Asians in London. *Psychol. Med.* 1997;27: 791–798.

51. Van Os J, Castle DJ, Takei N, et al. Psychotic illness in ethnic minorities: Clarification from the 1991 census. *Psychol. Med.* 1996;26:203–208.

52. Hickling FW, Robertson-Hickling H, Hutchinson G. Caribbean migration and mental health. In: Hickling FW, Sorel E, eds. *Images of Psychiatry in the Caribbean.* Department of Community Health and Psychiatry, Mona; 2005:153–178.

53. Sharpley M, Hutchinson G, McKenzie K, et al. Understanding the excess of psychosis among the African-Caribbean population in England: Review of current hypotheses. Br J Psychiatry Suppl. 2001;40:s60–s68.

54. Harrison G, Glazebrook C, Brewin J, et al. Increased incidence of psychotic disorders in migrants from the Caribbean to the United Kingdom. *Psychological Medicine*. 1997;27:799–806.

55. Minsky S, Vega WA, Miskimen T, et al. Diagnostic patterns in Latino, African American, and European American psychiatric patients. *Arch Gen Psychiatry*. 2003;60:637–644.

56. Bengi-Arslan L, Verhulst FC, Crijnen AAM. Prevalence and determinants of minor psychiatric disorder in Turkish immigrants living in the Netherlands. *Social Psychiatry and Psychiatric Epidemiology*. 2002;37(3):118.

57. Llacer A, Del Amo J, Garcia-Fulgueiras A, et al. Discrimination and mental health in Ecuadorian immigrants in Spain. *Epidemiol Community Health*. 2009;63(9):766–772.

58. Qureshi A, Collazos F, Sobradiel N, et al. Epidemiology of psychiatric morbidity among migrants compared to native born population in Spain: A controlled study. *General Hospital Psychiatry*. 2013;35(1).

59. Escobar JI. Guía de consulta de los criterios Diagnósticos del DSM-5: Spanish edition of the Desk Reference to the Diagnostic Criteria from DSM-5. *American Journal of Psychiatry*. 2014;171:587–588.

60. Escobar JI, Lopez C. The classification of mental disorders in the international classification of diseases. In: Sadock BJ, Sadock VA, Ruiz, P., eds. *Kaplan and Sadock's Comprehensive Textbook of Psychiatry*. 10th ed. Philadelphia: Wolters Kluwer; 2017.

61. Lewis Fernandez R, Aggarwal N, Baarnhielm S, et al. Operationalizing cultural formulation for DSM-5. *Psychiatry: Interpersonal and Biological Processes*. 2014;77(2):130–154.

62. Escobar JI, and Marin H. Present and future of classification systems for mental disorders. In: Sadock BJ, Sadock VA, Ruiz, P., eds. *Kaplan and Sadock's Comprehensive Textbook of Psychiatry*. 10th ed. Philadelphia: Wolters Kluwer; 2017.

63. First MB. Harmonization of ICD-11 and DSM-V: Opportunities and challenges. *Br J Psychiatry*. 2009;195:382–390.

64. Jablensky A. Towards ICD-11 and DSM-V: Issues beyond "harmonization." *Br J Psychiatry*. 2009;195:379–381.

65. Reed GM, First MB, Kogan C., et al. Innovations and changes in the ICD-11 classification of mental, behavioral, and neurodevelopmental disorders. *World Psychiatry*. 2019;18:3–19.

66. Ozamiz N, Ortiz Jauregui A, Guimon J, Escobar JI. Personality disorders in the Basque region of Spain: Applicability of DSM-5's alternative criteria for personality disorders. *American Journal of Psychiatry*. 2016;173(8):769–770.

67. Sackett DL, Rosenberg WM, Gray JA, et al. Evidence based medicine: What it is and what it isn't. *BMJ*. 1996;312:71–72.

68. Chang S, Lee TH. Beyond evidence-based medicine. *New England Journal of Medicine*. 2018;379:1983–1985.

69. Barth J, Munder T, Gerger H, et al. Comparative efficacy of seven psychotherapeutic interventions for patients with depression: A network meta-analysis. *PLoS Med.* 2013;10(5):e1001454. doi:10.1371/journal.pmed.1001454.

70. Psychotherapy helps depression. *Nature.* 2013;49:385. doi:1038/499383e.

71. Weissman MM, Markowitz JC, Klerman GL. *The Guide to Interpersonal Psychotherapy.* Oxford: Oxford University Press; 2017.

72. WHO. Group Interpersonal Therapy (IPT) for Depression: WHO Generic Field Trial. Version 1.0. Geneva: World Health Organization and Columbia University; 2016.

73. Weissman MM. Psychotherapy: A paradox. *Am J Psychiatry.* 2013;170(7):712–715.

74. Bolton P, Bass J, Neugebauer R, et al. Group interpersonal psychotherapy for depression in rural Uganda: A randomized controlled trial. *JAMA.* 2003;289(23):3117–3124.

75. Patel V, Weiss HA, Chowdhary N, et al. Effectiveness of an intervention led by lay health counsellors for depressive and anxiety disorders in primary care in Goa, India (MANAS): A cluster randomized controlled trial. *Lancet.* 2010;18:376(9785):2086–2095. Epub Dec 13.

76. Rahman A, Malik A, Sikander S, et al. Cognitive behavior therapy–based intervention by community health workers for mothers with depression and their infants in rural Pakistan: A cluster-randomized controlled trial. *Lancet.* 2008;13:372(9642):902–909.

77. Sumathipala A, Hewege S, Hanwella R, et al. Randomized controlled trial of cognitive behavior therapy for repeated consultations for medically unexplained complaints: A feasibility study in Sri Lanka. *Psychol. Med.* 2000;30(4):747–757.

78. Alarcon RD. Mental health and mental health care in Latin America. *World Psychiatry.* 2003;2(1):54–56.

79. Rojas MG, Solis J, Castillo G, et al. Treatment of postnatal depression in low-income mothers in primary-care clinics in Santiago, Chile: A randomised controlled trial. *Lancet.* 2007;370:1629–1637).

80. Calderon J, Rojas G. Integration of mental health into primary care: A Chilean perspective on a global challenge. *BJPsych Int.* 2016;13(1):20–21.

81. Marin H, Escobar JI. Special issues in the psychopharmacological management of Hispanic patients. *Psychopharmacology Bulletin.* 2001;35(4):197–212.

82. Escobar JI, Tuason VB. Antidepressant agents: A cross-cultural study. *Psychopharmacology Bulletin.* 1980;16(3):49–52.

83. Escobar JI, Gomez J, Tuason VB. Depressive phenomenology in North American and South American patients. *American Journal of Psychiatry.* 1983;140(1):47–51.

2 · LOOKING AT CULTURAL ASPECTS OF GLOBAL MENTAL HEALTH

The Culturally Infused Engagement Model in Latin American and Asian Populations

MIWA YASUI AND KATHLEEN J. POTTICK

The World Health Organization's Mental Health Action Plan (2013–2020) reported a large, worrisome gap worldwide between the need for treatment and its provision.[1] Scarce health-system resources, inadequate policy guidelines, underdeveloped mental health surveillance methods, and an overreliance on hospitalization responses over community-based ones compromise the development of an integrated approach to identifying and treating mental health problems. Coupled with discrimination and stigmatization of mental health problems, these persistent factors undermine the ability of children and families to receive appropriate and necessary care.[1] Around the globe, disparities in treatment use are especially pronounced in low- and middle-income countries, with between 76 percent and 85 percent of people with serious mental disorders receiving no treatment at all. Though the treatment gap is smaller in high-income countries (35 percent to 50 percent), the problem remains ubiquitous.[1]

In the United States, racial and ethnic disparities in mental-health service use and treatment outcomes are an unrelenting and unresolved challenge, despite decades of attention to the issue. In the multicultural context of the United States, ethnic and racial minority children and families continue to be less likely to access mental health services than their mainstream counterparts[2] and are more likely to delay seeking treatment and to drop out of treatment.[3-6] Researchers have found that racial and ethnic disparities in the use of and benefit from mental health services often result from logistical barriers,[7] as well as pressures of poverty and racism,[8] stigma associated to receiving mental health care,[9] and lack of knowledge about mental health.[6] Psychological and sociocultural stressors, such as discrimination, acculturation, and cultural isolation, add to the risk for mental health problems while simultaneously reducing the chances that mental health help will be sought by racial and ethnic minority children and families.[4,10] In the United States and across the globe, the increased risk for mental health problems coupled with inadequate provision or use of treatments and services is costly to children, families, and communities, limiting their life chances and compromising their social and emotional well-being and their ability to assume productive life roles.

Culture plays a central role in understanding mental health problems and devising approaches for their proper management.[11] As culture contextualizes mental health problems, it is the linchpin for globally relevant scholarship to make sense of variations in how mental health issues and their treatment are conceptualized by different racial and ethnic groups. While there is some debate about its definition, most scholars define culture as an intergenerationally transmitted system of meanings that encompasses values, beliefs, and expectations, including traditions, customs, and practices shared by a group or groups of people.[12] Culture has the stability to define the boundary of a group, as well as the flexibility to be transformed in everyday experience. Culture shapes the very meaning of health and approaches to healing at multiple levels—from the individual's beliefs, attitudes, and practices, to the broader expectations, beliefs, and practices of families, communities, and cultures, involving complex challenges of navigating individual, familial, and culturally derived sets of beliefs, attitudes, and practices. There is a dearth of empirical research specifying how ethnic and cultural factors influence the treatment engagement process.[13,14] Thus, better understanding of cultural and contextual factors specific to mental-health service use may be critical in identifying key mechanisms of treatment engagement that can enhance care for different ethnic groups of children and families.

In this chapter, we call for a paradigm shift in the way that mental health is studied and practiced with ethnic minority and immigrant children and families in the United States, and by corollary, with different ethnic groups in their home countries. In earlier work, we developed the Culturally Infused Engagement (CIE) model[15] to provide an urgently needed framework for a new conceptualization of engagement, going from current approaches that limit engagement to a process of treatment and participation, to a broader one that begins at problem recognition and expressions of distress. The CIE model builds on several theoretical models of mental health from the disciplines of medical anthropology, cultural psychiatry, health studies, social psychology, and mental health that address the integral nature of culture in the mental health and its healing approaches. These models include (a) the Socio-Cultural Framework for the study of Health Service Disparities (SCF-HSD)[13] that illustrates multilevel influences of culture that influence the utilization of mental health services; (b) the mental health help-seeking framework[14] that describes how individuals progress through stages of problem recognition to engagement in healing; (c) Kleinman's[16] Explanatory Models of Illness, a central foundation of cultural conceptualizations of mental illness or mental distress that encompasses personal and social meanings of the illness experience and approaches of healing and treatment; and (d) the Theory of Planned Behavior model,[17] which represents internal mechanisms of help-seeking intentions and actions that guide diverse populations' processes of engaging in treatment.

In our previous work, we applied the CIE model in a targeted review of 119 available clinical assessment instruments keyed to the CIE to identify items that could capture the multidimensional and developmental processes involved in mental health detection and the help-seeking experiences of multiple ethnic minority and immigrant populations. In the course of that review, we showed that Western definitions of illness and related treatments may not be useful for ethnic minority and immigrant children and families in the United States, whose perspectives are shaped by unique cultural beliefs, values, practices, and norms affecting how illness is characterized and treatment is understood. For ethnic minority and immigrant families, expressions of distress and their meaning were embedded in multiple levels of a person's life, including individual beliefs, attitudes, and practices, as well as family expectations, values and practices, community norms, and worldviews.[14,18,19] These elements dictated the process of clinical engagement, starting at the initial stage of help-seeking (recognizing a problem and finding help for it) and then participation in treatment (attending meetings or sessions). To assume inaccurately that ethnic minorities and immigrants (1) understand and accept the concept of "mental health" in the mainstream culture, (2) recognize their problems as mental health problems, and (3) perceive mental health services as appropriate helping solutions may significantly compromise effective outreach and service delivery.

Our new model, Culturally Infused Engagement (CIE),[15] is used to examine how culture influences identification of mental health problems and attitudes toward mental health help and helpers. In this chapter, we will focus primarily on the Latino/a or Hispanic (hereafter, Latino) population, which is the main focus of this book, but we will also highlight Asian populations, the fastest-growing group in the United States.[20] These ethnic groups also underutilize mental health services.[21,22] The CIE can provide insight into globally relevant opportunities for understanding culturally infused engagement approaches at the clinical level for them. By applying this multidimensional and developmental process model, we may help to unmask important mechanisms of ethnic disparities in service utilization and provide guidance to clinicians not only in the United States but globally. First, we briefly provide a contemporary perspective on culture and its influence on the trajectory of engagement in mental health services for culturally diverse individuals. Second, we describe the CIE model. Third, we identify what is known about engagement processes for Latino populations. Fourth, we describe the literature on engagement for Asian populations. Finally, we synthesize our findings, discussing their implications for clinical innovation.

THE ARCHITECTURE OF HELP-SEEKING FOR ETHNICALLY DIVERSE INDIVIDUALS AND FAMILIES

The Culturally Infused Engagement (CIE) model is a comprehensive model of the help-seeking process that illustrates how cultural and contextual influences from multiple systemic levels imbue the ecological context of ethnically diverse individuals and families. It captures how the explanatory models of mental illness that are purported by various systems and relationships (e.g., family member, community, culture) may critically shape the trajectory of treatment engagement for ethnically diverse individuals and families. While ethnically diverse individuals and families may endorse specific, unique values, beliefs, and practices regarding mental health and help-seeking, values, beliefs, and practices also interact with explanatory models and mechanisms of help-seeking at the meso-level (i.e., ethnic community, church, school, and neighborhood). Influences of macro-level factors, such as discrimination or the U.S. mainstream culture (e.g., media exposure on mental health), also directly or indirectly shape ethnically diverse individuals and families' understanding of mental distress and illness, and hence, their treatment engagement. The infusion of these multifaceted influences is played out at the individual level as unique explanatory models of illness.

The explanatory model serves as a blueprint that weaves together the beliefs, intentions, and behavioral and emotional responses and reveals how the ethnically diverse individual understands the lived experience of illness. The model encompasses how the ethnically diverse individual (a) conceptualizes distress, which constitutes his or her understanding of the illness cause, course, identity, and illness experience; and (b) responds to the mental illness/distress (i.e., healing approaches). The way in which the ethnically diverse individual conceives his or her mental distress is central to the stage of problem recognition. It involves a multidimensional view of distress: (1) the understanding of the causes (e.g., psychological, biological, supernatural); (2) the very expressions (e.g., idioms) of distress; (3) the identity of the illness, which is interlaced with causal beliefs; and (4) the personal meanings that the ethnically diverse individual derives from his or her illness experience. The meaning of the illness experience is molded by (i) beliefs of the internal traits and characteristics of the individual with the illness, (ii) behavioral beliefs about mental distress (i.e., its expected outcomes), and (iii) agency beliefs (i.e., perceived control over the illness or distress) that encompass the effect of external barriers (e.g., lack of insurance, transportation issues, lack of childcare) on the lived illness experience. Simultaneously, these individualized beliefs are affected by perceived norms (the perceived meanings of the illness or distress for others) that further determine the meaning of the individual's lived experience of illness within broader sociocultural contexts (see figure 2.1). Thus, an individual's response to the illness experience in both help-seeking and treatment participation is the result of the integration of individualized beliefs and perceived norms that serve as the basis for the seeking of relevant methods of healing.

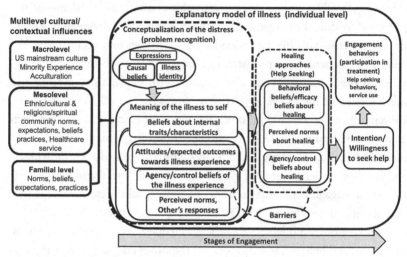

FIGURE 2.1. The Culturally Infused Engagement (CIE) model. Reprinted by permission from Springer: Yasui M, Pottick KJ, Chen Y. Conceptualizing culturally infused engagement and its measurement for ethnic minority and immigrant children and families. *Clin Child Fam Psychol Rev.* 2017; 20(3):250–332.

Our earlier work examined the measures for the developmental and help-seeking processes from the CIE model on ethnic minority and immigrant children and families in the United States. This chapter focuses on the complex and unique architecture of help-seeking processes among Latino and Asian individuals and families. The review relies on many studies conducted in Spanish-speaking and Asian countries, as well as in the United States. Thus, the chapter can provide new information to understand experiences of immigrant populations in the United States, as well as populations in the home countries. It illustrates the practical utility of this perspective to provide insight into expressions of distress, meaning of the illness experience, help-seeking, and treatment participation for these individuals and families to inform clinical and programmatic solutions to mental health disparities for them. While this chapter focuses primarily on Latinos and Asians, the model can be applied to other ethnically diverse individuals and families to yield new, valuable information for global practice. While this model has been used primarily in mental health settings in the United States, it should work optimally in well-integrated systems that offer mental health embedded in primary care services. We believe it can also be used successfully in a primary care context globally, given the shortage of mental health specialists.

EXAMINING THE LITERATURE ON CULTURE AND MENTAL HEALTH SERVICES FOR LATINOS AND ASIANS

Our literature review was guided by a scoping approach, which involves a number of searches that address a broad set of questions rather than a single search targeted to one primary question. This type of approach is particularly well suited for areas of inquiry that are being newly generated. It uses a qualitative synthesis of extant studies to appraise the conceptual boundaries of a heterogeneous field and to identify its size and scope.[23] Our chapter scopes the available evidence that examines the application of the CIE model for Asian and Latino populations globally. We searched for keywords that mapped onto each of the CIE domains specific to the population (i.e., Asian, Latino). A computerized literature search using PsychINFO, ERIC, Ingenta Connect, Google Scholar, JSTOR, and PubMed databases was conducted for relevant articles between 1960 and 2018. The keywords used for the review of the literature included the following: culture, Asian, Latino, immigrant, ethnic minority, culturally bound syndromes, somatic distress, explanatory models of illness, mental health, emotional distress, idioms of distress, mental health beliefs, causal beliefs, stigma, help-seeking, mental health services, and mental health treatment. In addition, we included relevant articles from a prior literature review where we proposed the CIE model.[15] Articles are included in this chapter if they (a) reported on Latino or Asian samples and (b) addressed at least one of the CIE dimensions in study findings. It is important to note that our review uses racial and ethnic categories as they are reported in existing studies, understanding that they may be culturally, contextually, and geographically defined. We refer to them solely in reporting the descriptions of previous articles. A total of 201 articles were reviewed, of which 125 were selected for this chapter. Our findings are presented for each group through the conceptual lens of the CIE dimensions, specifying what is known about their help-seeking processes.

CULTURALLY INFUSED ENGAGEMENT PROCESSES FOR LATINOS

Conceptualization of the Distress (Problem Recognition)

Expressing distress. Latinos are a heterogeneous group from socioeconomic, racial, and cultural perspectives. Most studies on illness perception and mental health treatment of Latinos have been done in immigrant populations in the United States, and we do not know if these results can be extrapolated to the native cultures. In general, studies within and outside the United States have suggested that Latino individuals with mental health problems show a tendency to present to medical and mental health service settings exhibiting physical rather than psychological symptoms. Latinos have also been reported to be more likely to endorse somatic symptoms as idioms of distress and to report different symptom clusters compared to their White non-Hispanic counterparts. Specifically, when conventional measures of psychological distress such as depression, anxiety, ADHD, and others are used, Latinos are found to report varying thresholds of symptom severity as well as a constellation of associated physical symptoms compared to their White non-Hispanic counterparts.[24-26] For example, in a study by Contreras and colleagues,[27] Latino college students scored higher than White non-Hispanic students on physiological symptoms of depression and anxiety (e.g., numbness, wobbliness, inability to relax, dizziness, hands trembling) as measured by the Beck Depression Inventory[28] and the Beck Anxiety Inventory.[29] Crain and colleagues[30] found that the most common mental health symptoms reported by Latino farmworkers were general lethargy or malaise and inability to relax. This sense of malaise and nervousness that was described as *los nervios* was the most prevalent symptom endorsed by Latino college students and working poor Latinos.[31]

Somatic symptoms. The salience of somatic symptoms as indicators of distress has also been well documented in studies on the culturally bound syndrome *ataque de nervios,* which involves a constellation of somatic symptoms that range from heart palpitations, shaking or trembling, rising heat, and numbness, and these are often accompanied by behaviors such as crying, shouting, and aggression.[32,33] According to Guarnaccia and colleagues,[32] ataque de nervios is understood as a culturally determined response to acute stressful circumstances (e.g., funerals, accidents, or family conflict). Studies report the overlap of ataque de nervios with mental disorders including panic disorder, anxiety, and depression.[34,35] However, Latinos identify ataque de nervios as a cultural expression of distress that is distinct from mental disorders and in fact express varying symptom presentations.[36]

Cultural idioms of distress. Lewis-Fernandez and colleagues[37] point out that the culturally specific manifestations of mental distress are captured in the range of cultural idioms of distress that are often reported by Latinos. In addition to ataque de nervios, the cultural idioms of *estar nervioso* (which reflects a condition of being nervous since childhood) and *padecer de los nervios* (suffering from nerves) are frequently used to illustrate the distress that arises from stress and hardships.[37,38] Further, such experiences as *viendo celejaes* (seeing shadows) or *sentir una presencia* (feeling there is a presence) constitute a number of the auditory, tactile, or visual experiences that are often triggered by stress among Latinos.[37] Other culturally bound syndromes have been also described, starting with *el duende* (the ghost) in Latin America.[39] Also, certain spiritual folk traditions influence symptom presentation.[40]

More recent reviews of these culture-bound syndromes include syndromes such as *susto* (fright), which involves symptoms of restlessness, loss of weight and motivation, and listlessness; *mal de ojo* (evil eye), a condition that involves several somatic symptoms such as severe headaches, insomnia, and fever, as well as behaviors including weeping and fretfulness; and *empacho* (indigestion or gastrointestinal infection), which consists of stomach pains.[41]

This unique influence of culture not only shapes symptom expression but also determines the very thresholds of distress among Latinos. Bridges and colleagues[42] found that Latino patients endorsed lower psychiatric distress and that clinicians rated them with higher global assessment of functioning compared to non-Latino White patients. In another study, which examined symptoms of ADHD among children, Latino parents tended to rate hyperactive-impulsive behaviors as developmentally normative.[43] These findings may suggest that Latinos are more likely to perceive distress as nonproblematic because it is considered to be part of the normative experience of life as an immigrant who is buffeted by the pressures of poverty, family separation, and challenging work conditions.[34,43] However, studies have also reported an opposite trend by which Latino participants were more likely to overendorse symptoms, particularly symptoms related to PTSD.[44,45] Overendorsement of symptoms was also found among those who strongly adhered to cultural values and native traditions.[46,47]

The complexity surrounding the identification of mental distress (i.e., the way symptoms are regarded as indicators of distress thresholds) brings to light the need to consider the adequacy of existing clinical assessments in capturing the distress experiences of Latinos[48] and to look carefully at the implications of these phenomena for clinical practice.

Causal beliefs. Review of the literature indicated that causal beliefs of mental illness and distress were directly linked to how Latinos responded in their illness experience. Latinos are found to attribute mental illness and distress to a range of causes that include spiritual or supernatural forces (e.g., God, ghosts, spirits, luck, magic), fate or destiny, contextual stressors, and relationship problems.

De la Cancela and Martinez[49] report that Latino folk systems and religious views are a dominant influence on the beliefs that mental distress and illness are caused by actions of supernatural forces or the will of God. Caplan and colleagues[50] also found that spiritual factors such as lack of faith, punishment from God, the evil eye, and witchcraft or spells were identified as notable causes of depression among Dominican, Colombian, and Ecuadorian immigrants. Other studies, similarly, have found that Latinos attribute severe mental distress to evil spirits or spells.[40,51]

Relational strife was also identified as a major cause of mental distress among Latinos. Studies suggest that Latinos attribute marital problems and familial strife as the main causes of *nervios* (nerves) among individuals.[31,52] Falicov[53] notes that Latinos believe that negative social relations that elicit envy or revenge are the causes of attacks of *mal de ojo* (evil eye), and that *empacho* (indigestion) is caused by being forced to eat foods by another or accepting food offered by others out of politeness despite not being hungry. Caplan and colleagues[54] found that relational trauma, including domestic violence, abuse, and loss of loved ones, was the most cited reason for depression among Dominican, Colombian, and Ecuadorian immigrants. Cabassa and colleagues[55] noted that social dimensions (e.g., domestic violence, loss of a loved one, caregiving problems) were identified as central causes of depression among low-income Latinos.

Relatedly, fatalism, a cultural belief that individuals have no power or control over their lives, and that external forces determine the outcome of health and illness,[40,56,57] is associated with beliefs that attribute luck or destiny or God's will as the cause of mental distress and illness.

Finally, sociocultural stressors such as racial discrimination and acculturative stress were identified by Latino immigrant populations as causes of mental distress. Chapman and Stein[58] found that Latino parents identified racism and immigrant status as causes of youths' problem behaviors, as illus-trated by a participant: "Since we are immigrants, they make us feel that we are third-class citizens. A person from a third class and that we are not worth the same as someone from here. These things could affect her [the girl in the scenario]. The racism that exists between races here . . ."[p278]

Illness Identity and Characteristics Associated with Individuals with the Illness

The understanding of how distress and mental illness concepts are construed provides an essential frame for examining the ways in which individuals expe-rience and make meaning of their distress. Studies suggest that Latinos draw a distinction between mental illness and mental distress, where the for-mer is associated with severe dysfunction or disability and the latter is asso-ciated with culturally appropriate responses to family and environmental stressors. For example, Mexican participants in a study by Rogers and Gallegos[59] attributed poor mental health to "being crazy" or *loco*. Partici-pants expressed poor mental health as "being sick in the head" or "losing themselves," which was associated with irrational behaviors and abnormal-ity in cognitive functions. Kaltman and colleagues[60] found that low-income immigrant women from Central America, South America, and Mexico were likely to link mental health terminology with expressions such as "being *loco* (crazy), *pasado* (lapsed) or *transtornadito* (deranged)"; and further, these beliefs influenced women's negative attitudes towards seeking mental health services. As an example, a participant in this study described people with mental illness as "those who try to hurt themselves, pull out their hair, act hysterically, and do not have self-control."[60 (p88)]

The Meaning of the Illness Experience

As described as part of the CIE model, the illness experience is determined by how individuals conceptualize their mental distress. Existing literature on the illness experience of some Latino groups in the United States reveals two perspectives of mental distress: (1) the interpretation of distress as mental illness, and (2) the explanation of distress as culturally normative phenom-ena. These studies have revealed the centrality of the culture in describing the ways Latinos perceived and responded to their experiences of mental distress. In particular, studies highlight the influence of cultural values such as *familismo*, *marianismo*, and *machismo*, as well as the importance of self-reliance, for understanding how social norms influence Latinos' individual expectations and sense of agency (i.e., perceived control, self-efficacy) regarding their illness experience. What seems striking is how these two domains are intertwined in the ways Latinos approach their illness experience.

Attitudes, expectations, and agency beliefs when distress is construed as mental illness. Latino cultural values play a dominant role in shaping individual-level expectations and agency beliefs about the illness experience. For example, the construct of machismo may impede Latino males' inclination to acknowledge their mental illness or motivate them to attempt to try to cope with their symptoms alone rather than seek help, due to fears of being seen as having a weak character.[61,62] For females, the notion of self-sacrifice emphasized in the cultural value of marianismo may pressure women to cope with severe mental health symptoms alone or with the family, and discourage seeking outside treatment.[63] Moreover, the Latino cultural value of familismo, defined as a "sense of obligation to, and connectedness with one's immediate and extended family,"[64(p259)] influences their view of mental illness. Familismo's strong emphasis on family cohesion may deter individuals from disclosing their mental illness to family members due to fears of being perceived as weak, crazy, or a burden.[65]

Fatalism has been related to the lower likelihood seen among Latinos to seek help for their mental distress, resulting in a resignation of efforts to change or improve their condition.[25,26] This resignation to external forces dictates individuals' agency beliefs regarding their illness experience, as illustrated in a participant's quote from a study by Martinez-Tyson and colleagues:[66] "No one can prevent it. Depression happens because of problems. At least right now as things are, people get depressed because they don't have a job. People look for work and there are no jobs, so people get depressed. The bills and everything piling up."[(p1294)]

Social norms for when distress is construed as mental illness. Literature on mental illness highlights public stigma as the shared negative beliefs and attitudes that prompt others to reject, avoid, and discriminate against persons with mental illness.[67,68] This potential stigma remains a major concern for people with mental illness within Latino communities. Latinos' cultural conceptualizations of individuals with mental illness as *loco* or crazy or weak[60,69] strongly influence the social responses of others toward individuals with mental illness. Studies indicate that Latinos fear a range of social responses—either from their ethnic community or family—including being excluded, ignored, made fun of, or harassed by others.[60,66] Concerns regarding the repercussions of stigma extended across a variety of contexts—from fears of bringing shame on the family,[70] to worries about being negatively evaluated in the workplace,[65,71] to concerns of being talked about in one's community.[72,73] Highlighting the impact of social stigma at the larger community level, one study also reported that an attitude of indifference was a common response of the community to individuals with mental illness.[66] As a result, Latino individuals with mental illness are found to respond to social stigma by withholding information about their mental illness or refusing to seek help outside of the family.[74]

Latino cultural values are also closely tied to some of the social stigma beliefs identified in the literature. For example, the traditional cultural gender role of machismo emphasizes qualities such as masculinity, male dominance, responsibility as the protector of the family, and physical strength.[75,76] This cultural expectation for Latino males to be strong can facilitate social attitudes that pressure Latino males to deny or minimize mental health symptoms, despite evident distress.[69,77] Moreover, familismo's emphasis on family cohesion may increase stigmatizing attitudes and responses within the family, particularly when social stigma beliefs are adopted by family members.[65]

The strong influence of social stigma is also related to Latinos' endorsement of courtesy stigma, which is the extension of the stigma to close others such as family and friends. For example, Magana and colleagues[78] report that Latino caregivers of adults with schizophrenia were less likely to talk to others about family members with mental illness or seek outside support because of the stigma associated with the mental illness. Marques and Ramirez Garcia[79] found that caregivers of Latinos with severe mental illness tended to delay help-seeking because of concerns about how their family would be viewed by others, as well as shame about mental illness.

Attitudes, expectations, and agency beliefs when distress is consonant to cultural views of distress. Across several studies, the core cultural value of familismo was identified as a central value that directed Latinos' expectations and sense of agency over their illness experience. The emphasis of familismo on the maintenance of family cohesion, through supporting and sacrificing for the family, even over personal or individual needs and goals,[80-82] appeared to impact how individuals approached their distress. Familismo was found to influence the help-seeking pathways of Latinos— how individuals may acknowledge their distress, disclose problems to others, and select sources of help or ways to cope, [77,83] suggesting the centrality of familial norms and expectations in shaping individuals' views of their illness experience.

Several studies note how consideration of familial responses and expectations determined an individual's own understanding and reaction to distress. For example, Ishikawa and colleagues[77] reported that in their study of Latino men and women, the dismissal of suffering by family members influenced individuals to interpret their distress as something that did not merit attention, which resulted in the denial or minimization of their own distress. Thus, the minimization of distress by family members leads individuals to endorse self-reliance, or, as described by Ortega and Alegria,[84] the preference "to solve their emotional problems on their own."(p133) While this notion of self-reliance may appear to counter the concept of familismo, studies indicate that Latinos perceive seeking support or disclosing distress as prioritizing an individual's problem and needs, and further, bringing shame on the family.[85,86] In this way, heeding familial norms and expectations emerged as the driving force behind individuals developing their own expectations and responses to distress (i.e., self-reliance).

The cultural value of marianismo, which requires women to emulate the Virgin Mary by sacrificing their own needs for their family and fulfill major caregiving roles of emotional and instrumental support,[87-89] encourages women to cope with their own distress internally and alone.[90] For example, Latina participants are reported to cope with depression individually through spiritual practices, keeping busy, or self-medicating with herbs and other home remedies.[59,91,92]

Social norms when distress is consonant to cultural views of distress. Familismo plays an instrumental role in helping Latino individuals cope with mental distress, particularly when there is a shared understanding and acknowledgment of the distress by salient norm groups such as family members. Ishikawa and colleagues[77] found that Latinos reported the importance of familial support in helping them cope with their mental distress. A quote from one of the participants in their study illustrates the significance of the family: "My family immediately . . . came down . . . and they like talked to me and stuff, which really helped. . . . I spent a month at home, which really, you know, I was able to focus again. I really needed that, to be sur- rounded by family and surrounded by people who understand, so I needed my community again, so once I was surrounded by my best friends, and like, my family again, that's when I calmed down, I was able to focus again."[77(p1563)]

Healing Approaches and Engagement in Help Seeking

The current evidence on the underutilization of mental health services among Latinos signals the dire need to understand the pathways to engagement, starting from conceptualization and moving to the illness experience as illus- trated in the CIE.

Seeking help from cultural sources. Latinos engage a variety of alternate help- seeking sources that are rooted in traditional or indigenous models of illness that link causes of mental illness and distress to supernatural, spiritual, and cultural elements. For example, healing approaches for the culturally bound syndrome *susto* (fright) may involve enlisting the help of *curanderos*, tradi- tional healers to help a person recapture his or her soul and return it to the body.[53] Latinos may also seek the help of sorcerers (*brujos, brujas*) or priests to counter the attacks of spiritual forces (e.g., devil, evil spirit, or witchcraft) that they believe are the causes of strong negative emotions (e.g., envy, anger, intense fear) or interpersonal conflict.[40] In addition, Latinos utilize herbs and plants that are also provided by traditional healers to treat illnesses in the body and mind.[93]

As mentioned earlier, social relationships are central informal sources of help for Latinos. Studies indicate that Latinos believe that receiving social support from family and spiritual or religious leaders reduces emotional dis- tress.[31,94] Addressing the mental distress within close relationships is per- ceived as sufficient in meeting the emotional and psychological needs of the individual and is often the first and foremost approach to help-seeking. Jen- kins[95] notes this central emphasis of family responsibility in response to mental distress and illness—that the family is the first line of healing and care—even in circumstances where the individual may struggle with severe mental illness. However, this emphasis on seeking support within close rela- tionships can delay or even interfere with the seeking of mental health ser- vices for severe mental distress.

Seeking help from mental health services. Existing literature on attitudes toward mental health services indicates that among Latinos, seeking mental health services and seeing a mental health professional are largely seen as practices that counter cultural norms and values. In general, Latinos view mental health services as a treatment option that is exclusively for individuals who exhibit extreme dysfunction,[77] and as a last option.[60] In particular, Latinos are found to approach the use of medication for treating mental illness with attitudes of distrust and skepticism. Studies indicate that Latinos believe that medication is unable to solve emotional problems, not appropriate for mental disorders, and even harmful.[60,62,97]

Attitudes toward seeking mental health services for distress or mental illness were also influenced by agency beliefs. Several barriers to seeking mental health services emerged from the literature, including low mental health literacy, logistical barriers such as transportation and finances, fears surrounding confidentiality, fears of stigma, and cultural values of self-reliance.

Several studies noted that low mental health literacy was reported by participants as a major barrier to mental health service use. For example, Kaltman and colleagues[60] found that uncertainty about what it means to go to a mental health provider was the most salient barrier for low-income Latino immigrant women. The lack of knowledge of what mental health services offered, where to find services, and how to use them was prevalent among Latinos, pointing to significant implications of low mental health literacy in treatment engagement.[60,66,78]

Logistical barriers were also cited across studies, particularly language barriers and immigration status. Studies have found that regardless of English proficiency levels, many Latinos report a preference for communicating health-related information in their native language.[100,101] Therapist ethnic and language match was highlighted as an important factor among Latinos particularly for counseling and psychotherapy services, as participants across studies noted concerns of not being able to speak openly and accurately about their problems and not being fully understood by their provider.[60,66,77] A number of studies also reported that fear of immigration issues had a negative impact on Latino participants' views of seeking mental health services. Fear of deportation was noted particularly for participants who were undocumented, as illustrated in a quote by a Colombian woman in the study by

Martinez-Tyson and colleagues[66]: "At least immigrant people, people without their documents, that makes them afraid, afraid of [getting help]." Finally, the cost of mental health care and the difficulty of transportation or access to services were also identified as significant barriers to mental health services use.[60,99]

Latino individuals' sense of agency in seeking mental health services was also affected by sociocultural barriers. As we have described, self-reliant attitudes that are associated with traditional cultural gender roles of machismo and marianismo are likely to deter individuals from seeking mental health services and instead lead them to cope with their mental health issues alone. Ortega and Alegria[84] found that among Puerto Ricans, individuals who reported higher self-reliant attitudes were 40 percent less likely to use mental health services. In addition, studies reported that mental health stigma beliefs elicited Latinos' fears about confidentiality and disclosing personal and sensitive information to an unknown stranger.[60] Such concerns were more elevated among Latinos who endorsed stronger familism than those with lower endorsements, highlighting the significant bearing Latino culture has on decisions on help-seeking.[62,79]

Across studies ranging from Latino youth to adults, negative attributions such as "crazy" or "*loco*" were associated with individuals who use mental health services, highlighting the prevailing effects of social stigma.[60,66,69] Studies noted that the reluctance to seek mental health services was related to fears regarding the consequences of stigma, including a lack of support from family and friends, lack of acceptance or rejection from others, and shame.[62,66] In this way, the beliefs and perceptions of the illness experience (i.e., being stigmatized) appear to play a critical role in how individuals determine whether to seek professional mental health help. The pervasiveness of social stigma on individuals was also reflected in self-stigmatizing views of individuals, by which some labeled themselves as crazy or weak.[60,66] For example, a participant in Kaltman and colleagues'[60] study noted, "It is like you have doubts and you say: could it be that I am crazy? You think that going to a psychiatrist is only for crazy people."(p89) This perception of mental health services as exclusive to individuals with extreme mental distress continues to be a considerable barrier for Latinos' engagement in formal mental health services.

CULTURALLY INFUSED ENGAGEMENT PROCESSES FOR ASIANS

Conceptualization of the Distress (Problem Recognition)

Expressing distress. Similar to Latinos, Asians are heterogeneous, consisting of a wide range of ethnic groups diverse in culture, country of origin, history, and, moreover, in language, that uniquely influence the ways in which individuals exhibit, experience, and make meaning of mental distress.[102] Within the United States, Asians are the fastest-growing racial group, yet the least engaged in utilizing mental health services.[103,104] While literature on mental health beliefs and service use has largely centered on Asian immigrants in the United States, we expand our review to Asians in the global context.

Somatic symptoms. Review of the literature suggests that Asians express and experience mental distress across a wide range, encompassing somatic or bodily symptoms, culturally specific distress, relational concerns, and psychological symptoms. Similar to our findings with Latinos, the use of somatic symptoms to describe distress was prominent across various Asian populations. In many cases, individuals would express their distress through presenting somatic symptoms, expressing cultural idioms or culturally specific distress. For example, Punjabis describe depression as a "sinking heart" (*dil ghirda hai*) and associate it with somatic symptoms of the heart and chest.[105] Hsiao and colleagues[106] found that among Chinese Australian patients, anxiety was explained as a restless heart or having a fast heartbeat (*hsin huang*) and classified as a physical illness rather than a mental health problem. Muecke[107] found that Southeast Asian refugees generally reported their distress through physical phenomena such as having either a "weak heart," which refers to having palpitations, dizziness, fainting, or feelings of panic, or a "weak nervous system," which encompasses headaches, difficulty concentrating, and malaise or fatigue. The use of somatic expressions of distress was also reported among youth. For example, Choi[108] found that Asian American adolescents tended to complain about physical problems when asked about their distress. They referred to symptoms such as headaches, stomach pain, muscle tension, weight loss, poor appetite, and decreased desire for sex.

These somatic expressions of psychological or emotional distress are guided by culturally specific norms and expectations. For example, among South Asians and Arabs, physical problems are viewed as legitimate and morally acceptable expressions of pain.[109] Further, cultural gender roles and expectations that associate masculinity with strength and control have been found to influence Asian Indian males' conceptualization of their illness as somatic or physical in origin rather than psychological.[110] For East and Southeast Asians, the influence of traditional Chinese medicine likely emphasizes the physical manifestations of distress, as it purports the integration of the body, spirit, and mind whereby physical organs are understood as the origin of somatic and psychological distress.[105,110] In fact, scholars note that traditional Chinese medicine holds an "unwillingness to differentiate between psychological and physiological functions,"[112(p101)] which suggests a central emphasis on physical indicators as relevant for both physical and mental well-being.

Somatic symptoms not only serve as salient indicators of distress, but they also reveal emotional and cognitive manifestations of distress that Asian individuals may not readily recognize or acknowledge. For example, the Korean culturally bound syndrome *hwabyung*, also known as "anger disease," is characterized by symptoms of panic, fear of impending death, dysphoric affect, and anger, together with a range of somatic symptoms including insomnia, fatigue, indigestion, lack of vital energy, heart palpitations, generalized aches and pains, a feeling of a mass in the epigastrium, labored breathing, and anorexia.[113(p846)] According to Pang,[114] hwabyung is the physical manifestation of "disappointments, sadness, miseries, hostilities, grudges and unfulfilled dreams and expectations" that are due to social and cultural pressures to maintain harmonious relationships. Among Arabs, cultural idioms and proverbs that refer to the body are used to describe emotional distress. For example, "My heart fell down" is a phrase used to describe fear, and "My eye is blind and my hand is short" illustrates a person's inability to confront personal problems.[115] Cambodians use various sayings that include functions of the body to indicate psychological distress, such as "My brain is spinning" (*wul khueu khabaal*), which means, "I am overwhelmed"; "arrived to my neck," which means, "I cannot take it anymore"; and "carrying a heavy load at the shoulder," which means, "I am overburdened with responsibility."[116]

In addition to somatic expressions, emotional distress was also often described in cognitive, behavioral, situational, or relational terms. For example, among Cambodians the phrase "thinking a lot" illustrates anxiety that stems from struggles with current problems (e.g., money problems and problems with children), traumatic events of the past (e.g., genocide), or separation from loved ones due to death or physical distance (e.g., with parents and siblings living in Cambodia).[116] Hsiao and colleagues[106] reported that Chinese Australian patients would refer to having a "suspicious illness," which described excessive worry and feelings of insecurity about health or interpersonal problems. Marsella and colleagues[117] found that the Japanese would use relational expressions to describe a depressed mood, such as "unable to get along with other people," instead of reporting feelings. Among Asian Indian immigrants, feelings of depression or sadness were referenced in regard to situations (e.g., being fed up with their situation or fed up with life[110]).

Causal beliefs. Causal attributions to mental distress and mental health among Asians indicated a holistic view of illness or distress that encompassed supernatural, contextual or situational, relational, personality or character, biological, and psychological factors. Across studies, Asian individuals reported distress as resulting from a combination of various factors rather than a singular cause.

Given the emphasis on somatic expression of distress, many Asians attributed physical or bodily factors as the cause of mental illness and distress. In particular, the influence of traditional Chinese medicine, which purports a close mind-body connection, was observed in the physiological explanations given for why an individual had mental distress or illness. Hsiao and colleagues106 found that among Chinese Australians, the imbalance of ying and yang was identified as the cause of symptoms of neurasthenia or schizophrenia; as described by one participant, "My body had too much yinhuo which caused my illness (schizophrenia)."[(p64)] This notion of disequilibrium in the body as a cause of mental distress is also shared among Cambodians in their understanding of koucharang or "thinking too much."[121] Moreover, studies revealed that East Asians, in addition to users of traditional Chinese medicine, also attached other physical causes to mental illness and distress, including the deficiency of specific vitamins, the presence of heavy metals in the body, allergies to foods, or metabolic abnormalities.[123] This highlights the predominant view of the body and mind as interconnected rather than distinct—a model of health that is favored among Asian cultures.

Beliefs in supernatural causes of mental distress and mental illness were prevalent across South Asians, Southeast Asians, and East Asians. Supernatural causes reported included the influence of God or gods, sin, spirits, destiny, yin and yang, and karma. For example, among Arabs, mental illness was perceived as due to spirits, the evil eye, or sorcery,[124] and healing or restoration was understood as an act of God or through the work of angels.[125] Studies indicate that Southeast Asians view emotional disturbance as due to the possession of spirits, black magic, evil spells, or bad karma accumulated by the individual's past misdeeds in life or lives.[107,126] For South Asians and Christian East Asians, mental illness was attributed to "God's will," thereby guiding the type of help-seeking sources individuals sought.[120,127] Across groups, there appears to be a shared view that the affliction of mental illness and distress is due to individuals' past moral transgressions (e.g., sin, bad action in previous life) or misdeeds on which supernatural forces then exert consequences.[120,123,127,128]

Contextual or situational causes of mental illness and mental distress were also identified among Asians. For example, Ying[111] found that participants identified external stress from immigration adjustment problems, social stressors common to immigrants such as unemployment and poverty, as major causes of the mental distress. Similarly, Asian American young adults noted the impact of discrimination and being 1.5-generation (individuals who immigrated at a young age) or second-generation (i.e., American born) immigrants as significant stressors that impacted mental health functioning.[129] This recognition of social stressors due to migration and living in a racially stratified society was particularly apparent among Asian immigrant populations.

Alongside situational factors, several studies highlighted the importance of interpersonal relationships in how Asian individuals conceptualized mental illness and distress. Difficulty in close relationships, particularly familial and marital relations, was cited across studies. For example, Anand and Cochrane[120] found that South Asian women identified marital violence and being trapped in an unhappy family as situations that caused emotional distress. Hsiao and colleagues[130] found that among their sample Chinese Australian patients and their caregivers, family conflict and disturbance of family harmony were cited as major sources of emotional distress and psychological imbalance. Relational difficulties between parents and children were also reported as causes of distress. These included parenting preference for boys over girls, parental pressure and expectations for children to succeed academically and pursue reputable career paths, and disagreements about parenting practices and child expectations.[119,129,130] The relevance that close interpersonal relationships have for Asians in their understanding of distress reflects the centrality of interdependence across Asian cultures.[131,132]

Finally, internal causes of distress included personality characteristics and excessive cognitive processes. For example, Phillips and colleagues[133] noted that Chinese participants were more likely to attribute personality problems as the cause of mental illness than other factors. Excessive thinking was also identified among East Asians and Southeast Asians. Yang and colleagues,[134] for example, reported that excessive thinking (xiang tai duo) was considered a precipitant to mental illness. Among Cambodian refugee adolescents, thinking too much was identified as a cause of mental distress.[121]

Illness Identity and Characteristics Associated with Individuals with the Illness

Similar to our findings for Latinos, conceptualizations of distress among Asians generally included beliefs about distress as a mental illness and beliefs associated with culturally determined notions of distress. Distress as a mental illness was largely categorized as a "mental problem" or "craziness," portraying dysfunction or abnormality as a characteristic of personal or emotional weakness.[118,119] This conceptualization of mental illness was linked with diagnostic mental health disorders such as schizophrenia and depression.

In contrast, distress in Asian cultures was often conceptualized through a holistic view that integrated the body, mind, spirit, and relational contexts.[106,120] Distress was perceived as an imbalance or disruption of integrated processes between these elements—thus, the restoration of such imbalance would result in healing and health.[118,121] Distress that was identified within a cultural framework was usually expressed via cultural idioms of distress or culturally specific symptoms and was not associated with mental illness.

Further, some studies found that among Asian groups, distress itself was not recognized or acknowledged, or individuals were confused at what the distress entailed. For example, in a study by Hsiao and colleagues,[106] a Chinese Australian patient describes his confusion regarding his distress: "I have never suffered from this illness and my family does not suffer from this illness either. So I do not know about this illness. I do not know whether or not this illness is a real illness."(p64) Relatedly in other studies, individuals would report being unsure of how to categorize the distress—whether it was a mental health problem or a "normal life problem."[122] This leads to amorphous conceptualizations of the distress (e.g., something is wrong) or the construal of the distress as another disease or illness—as described by a

Taiwanese parent on the grandparents' understanding of her child's problems: "They just keep asking my husband when he [the child with autism] will recover. They think it [autism] is like the flu or something."[123(p1328)]

Beliefs associated with individuals having mental health problems centered on negative characteristics or internal traits such as weakness, laziness, craziness, violence, and unpredictability. For example, Chinese patients with schizophrenia reported that even family members would view them as violent and unpredictable.[107] Among Arabs, personal weakness or craziness is often associated with individuals who display extreme emotional reactions or those who are considered mentally ill.[128] The notion of "a crazy person" was the most frequently associated characteristic for persons with mental illness among Chinese and Chinese immigrant populations,[106,118] highlighting the stigma associated with mental illness. Further, the conceptualization of dysfunction or deficit was also illustrated in the description of individuals with mental illness as having something missing or not working correctly.[112, 119]

Meaning of the Illness Experience

Attitudes, expectations, and agency beliefs when distress is construed as a mental illness. Studies with Asian populations reported that individuals with mental illness struggled with negative perceptions of themselves, which included seeing themselves as worthless, damaged, bad, or of low class.[106,112,118] Such internalization of stigma may be particularly pronounced among Asian cultures, as culturally incongruent displays of behaviors and emotional reactions oppose the cultural values of social conformity and emotional restraint.[135,136]

Across studies, culturally anchored stigma colored individuals' experiences of mental illness. For example, Frye and McGill[121] reported that Cambodian adolescents and their families perceived the onset of a psychiatric episode as extremely embarrassing, given the culture's emphasis on family solidarity and family management of aberrant behavior. Among South Asians, gendered perspectives also shaped how individuals perceived the illness experience. For example, Guzder and Krishna[137] note that for Asian Indian women, having mental illness reinforces traditional family and cultural views of women as inherently more vulnerable to madness, shame, guilt, and instability compared to men. Lee and colleagues[129] found that among Asian American young adults, the cultural taboo to talk openly about mental health issues resulted in people concealing their problems from others, neglecting or denying their mental distress, or refraining from seeking help from others due to the fear of being negatively labeled. Thus, for many Asian individuals, the social and cultural perceptions of mental illness likely diminish individuals' beliefs about their agency or self-efficacy and expected positive outcomes as a person with mental illness.[118]

Social norms for when distress is construed as a mental illness. The majority of the studies examining the experiences of mental illness among Asian groups reported the salience of public stigma—that is, shared negative beliefs and attitudes that prompt others to reject, avoid, and discriminate against persons with mental illness.[67,68] Overall, stigma from family members, the ethnic community, and individuals' culture were most cited, along with courtesy stigma (i.e., the stigma extended to close others such as family and friends).

In general, societal responses to individuals with mental illness emphasized greater social distance by which they would avoid, exclude, or reject persons with mental illness. Social responses by others ranged from rejection, avoidance, and poor treatment (e.g., blaming, condemning) by family members and friends, to broader community- and society-level responses such as losing employment or being ostracized from one's faith or ethnic community.[118,120,128,138] For example, Yang and colleagues[139] reported that Chinese Americans were more likely to have attitudes that endorsed social restrictions on individuals with mental illness such as discouraging being friends with, dating, getting married, or having children. For Chinese Americans in this study, genetic causes of mental illness appeared as a central factor for separation—illustrated by participants' endorsement of genetic screening or knowing the family history of mental illness of a potential marriage partner. Sun and colleagues[140] found that in China, family members of those with mental illness indicated greater preference for social distance compared to the general public, illustrating the stark impact of stigma even within the family network. Similarly, in Lee and colleagues' sample of Chinese families in Hong Kong,[129] family members reported despising or disliking the individual with mental illness. On the other hand, studies with Chinese and Southeast Asians noted that the fear of losing face due to mental health stigma also resulted in family members hiding individuals with mental illness within their family or concealing them from society until their symptoms were so severe that they needed hospitalization.[107,129,138]

The experience of mental illness also affects family members through courtesy stigma. For example, Chinese patients with schizophrenia reported that their family members experienced unfair treatment because of their association with the patient.[141-144] Among South Asians, having a family member with mental illness is associated with devaluing of economic and marriage prospects, increasing the likelihood of separation or divorce, or decreasing the leverage for obtaining a second wife.[128,145] While mental health stigma is universal, among Asians the link between the fear of losing "face" and mental health stigma is a central mark of culturally unique ways in which stigma manifests across cultures.

Attitudes, expectations, and agency beliefs when distress is consonant to cultural views of distress. Culture plays a salient role in determining individuals' notions of wellness and distress and how they approach their experiences of distress. For Arabs, the importance of their faith would deter individuals from disclosing or affirming thoughts about killing themselves because suicide is condemned and would be perceived as bad, weak, and disloyal.[128]

Relationships shape the very expectations of the illness experience. For example, Liu and colleagues[119] found that for Chinese and Vietnamese immigrants, expectations and beliefs of the illness experience are significantly shaped by Confucian values that emphasize role obligations, relational harmony, and interdependence. The threshold of when health becomes illness is often determined by whether individuals are able to control their distress to the extent that they are able to maintain harmony in social relationships and fulfill familial roles and obligations. This expectation is particularly prominent in the family context. For example, a father's inability to care for his family due to mental distress signifies a problem in Chinese culture, where men are expected to lead the household and raise the family. A quote by a participant in the study by Hsiao and colleagues[130] illustrates this: "Now his mother and I look after him. He cannot stand this. . . . He is a man so his self-esteem is very important. . . . Now he feels that he is a man but that he makes trouble for the family and so he feels sad and *nei jiu* (guilt)."[(p1002)] Lee and colleagues[129] also noted that as long as young Asian American adults were able to succeed academically or achieve high financial or social status, family members were not concerned by mental distress. In this way, fulfilling relational expectations appears to be a major indicator of health status among Asians.

Social norms when distress is consonant to cultural views of distress. For many Asians, individual-level expectations and attitudes of the illness experience may reflect broader societal and cultural norms. For example, among cultures such as the Chinese, Korean, Vietnamese, and Japanese, there is a strong influence of Confucian thought and values that emphasize suppressing emotion and exerting self-control.[146,147] This has shaped cultural and social norms that consider the expression of emotion and distress as countercultural, often resulting in stigmatizing or dismissing attitudes and behaviors toward individuals struggling with mental distress.[135,136] For example, Yasui[148] found that among Chinese immigrant youth and adults, expressions of distress by Chinese youth and young adults were met with dismissal, minimization, or even ridicule by members in the family and community.

Stigma. "Courtesy" stigma is particularly salient in Asian cultures that emphasize the family over than the individual. For example, Frye and McGill[121] found that Cambodian refugees had a significant concern for loss of face when family members were unable to be united in managing an individual's distress, particularly when the distress was expressed counter to cultural norms. Similarly, Mak and Cheung[143] found that caregivers of Chinese individuals with mental health problems reported strong concerns about maintaining face and upholding cultural norms regarding appropriate responses to distress.

Healing Approaches and Engagement in Help-Seeking

Seeking help from cultural sources. Literature revealed that the primary ways Asians deal or cope with mental distress involve culturally anchored healing approaches that include spiritual sources of healing, use of cultural remedies, and seeking interpersonal support within close networks, particularly within the family. Individuals' use of these healing approaches appeared to be closely tied to the causes they attribute to mental distress (i.e., seek a spiritual healer if the distress is caused by spirits). For the majority of Asians, culturally anchored approaches to healing or coping with distress are the primary means of help and are prioritized above seeking professional health and mental health services.[126,128,149]

Seeking spiritual or supernatural healing approaches emerged as a salient solution for many Asian groups. For example, Anand and Cochrane[120] found that for South Asian Muslim women, prayer was reported as the most effective way to cope with symptoms of depression or schizophrenia. In addition, traditional healers such as fortune-tellers, *khatib* (healers who help ward off evil spirits), and Koranic healers (healers who use the Koran, the Islamic scripture, to ward off evil spirits) are often utilized by Arabs who are struggling with mental health problems.[128] Somasundaram and colleagues[126] found that for Cambodian adults, the use of Buddhist prayers, meditation, and breathing exercises were effective in treating distress. Among the Chinese, herbal medicine, individual prayer or having a monk pray over the family, *feng shui*, and traditional Chinese medicine are common remedies for distress.[118] Shyu, Tsai, and Tsai[123] found that Taiwanese parents of autistic children engaged in a variety of supernatural sources of healing that included seeking fortune-tellers, requesting prayers from a monk, and changing the child's name. Moreover, in Chinese culture, traditional Chinese medicine has a strong influence in shaping conceptualizations of health, which is understood as the balance of yin and yang.[107] As a result, many seek the services of traditional Chinese medicine doctors on top of care from a primary care physician or mental health professional.[106,149]

For most Asians, the family serves as the initial help-seeking source for individuals in times of distress. Anand and Cochrane[120] note that in South Asian culture, priority is placed on the family when addressing mental health or personal needs. This was particularly important for women, who confided in family regarding struggles with depression. Frye and McGill[121] found that Cambodian refugee parents will recommend ways for their children to cope with depression and somatic distress that include engaging in meditation, forgetting sad thoughts through laughter and smiling, and avoiding alcohol. This notion of referring to the family for guidance in navigating distress was also illustrated in the study by Ying[111] in which Chinese immigrant participants identified relying on family and friends as the optimal response to distress. However, this emphasis on "family first" may also be driven by Asian families' fear of losing face and upholding family honor by keeping mental health problems within the family.[120,150]

Seeking help from mental health services. In contrast to cultural approaches to distress, mental health services are often the last resort for most Asian individuals. Phillips and colleagues[133] reported that Chinese families would go through multiple alternate treatments for a family member with mental illness before setting foot into a professional mental health service. Akutsu, Castillo, and Snowden[151] indicate that among Chinese, Japanese, Filipino, and Korean Americans, those who refer themselves to mental health services are likely to have already exhausted the resources and support available in their social networks.

The literature suggests several underlying reasons for the delay in seeking professional mental health services, including mental health stigma, causal beliefs of mental illness, mistrust of providers and services, and barriers to access. As mentioned earlier, among Asians stigma remains one of the primary barriers to engagement in mental health services. Individuals fear the repercussions of stigma resulting from seeking psychiatric or mental health care, particularly social exclusion or becoming an outcast in their community. For example, among South Asians, use of mental health services is associated with the loss of *izzat* or public honor, denial of marriage, and increased likelihood of separation or divorce.[128,152] Atkinson, Ponterott, and Sanchez[153] found that compared to Anglo American students, Vietnamese students endorse higher concerns of stigma associated with seeking psychological help. In fact, studies across Asian cultures demonstrate that shame and concerns regarding loss of face, particularly for the family, result in poor engagement in professional mental health services.[138,154,155]

In addition to stigma, another salient reason for delayed engagement in mental health services is the incongruence between Asians' explanatory models of illness and mental health services. In particular, the causes that Asian individuals attribute to mental distress are central in determining whether they seek professional services. For example, Shiekh and Furnham[156] reported that individuals who identified supernatural causes of mental health problems were more likely to have negative attitudes toward seeking professional help compared to those who endorsed Western physiological causes. Fung and Wong[157] also found that East and Southeast Asian immigrant and refugee women who identified supernatural factors as causes of mental illness reported higher negative attitudes toward professional mental health services than those who subscribed to a Western stress model. Moreover, because for many Asian cultures health is understood as an integration of the physical, mental, social, and spiritual, Western psychiatric explanations and treatments of mental health problems were frequently rejected.[106,130,158] Lee and colleagues[129] note that this discrepancy in conceptualizations of mental distress can result in individuals underidentifying the severity or even the presence of mental distress.

Related to stigma and discrepant explanatory models, Asians, like other ethnic minorities, are more likely to be mistrustful of professional mental health services. A paramount concern across various Asian groups was the fear that professionals would not maintain confidentiality.[118,120] This concern was elevated particularly if the professional was of the same ethnic background and shared the client's ethnic community.[120] Mistrust of mental health professionals also stemmed from apprehension and mistrust of biomedical treatment approaches to mental distress, which countered many Asian individuals' understanding of the cause of and care for mental distress.[107] In fact, a professional's endorsement of a biomedical view of mental health can be perceived as rejecting important cultural and religious values, which can increase client mistrust.[128,159]

Finally, studies revealed a range of barriers that impeded engagement in mental health services. Lack of understanding of the roles of mental health professionals and what services are available for mental illness and distress were noted for Asian immigrants in the United States and Australia.[160,161] Studies also indicated logistical barriers that included the lack of availability of bilingual and bicultural providers, lack of insurance, high cost of services, and problems with transportation as central reasons for Asian individuals' underutilization of mental health services in the United States.[118,162-164] On a structural level, concerns about racism and discrimination were raised by participants in several studies, suggesting that barriers at the social level also impeded Asians' engagement in mental health services.[118,164]

CONCLUSIONS AND DISCUSSION

The mental health services field continues to struggle to bring clarity to the nebulous concept of culture that clinicians face in their everyday practice and the ways it affects client engagement in mental health services and treatment responsiveness. This occurs despite the fact that far-reaching calls have been made for cultural competence in mental health service delivery.[165-167] This chapter highlighted the salient and multifaceted processes of engagement, stretching from how individuals conceptualize their distress and emotional problems to their perspectives on seeking help and participating in it. We apply the Culturally Infused Engagement (CIE) model[15] to Latino and Asian populations, known to underutilize services despite need, and are growing ethnic communities in the United States. This chapter is a novel examination of the CIE to assess differential engagement processes of groups from two different sociocultural backgrounds so it can begin unraveling the complex phenomenon of culturally infused engagement for ethnically diverse individuals and families. While we recognize that the CIE cannot fully address the cultural plurality of Latino and Asian individuals and families, the findings from the reviews and discussions included in our chapter suggest that the framework can flexibly identify ethnic and culturally specific influences relevant to engagement.

The CIE has multiple practical applications for clinical practice for Latinos and Asians. First, it can be used to prompt practicing clinicians to consider the complex influences of culture that affect client engagement. The dimensions identified in the CIE can inform clinicians in addressing multiple domains of engagement within the context of assessment and intervention. For example, our chapter reported that Latinos view distress such as insomnia, severe headaches, fright (*susto*) or the evil eye (*mal de ojo*), as normative and nonproblematic constellations of somatic symptoms that might otherwise be seen as mental health problems in Western diagnostic thinking. Among Asians, our chapter showed that causes of mental distress may be attributed to energy imbalance within the body (i.e., the flow of *ying* and *yang*) or moral failings of parents or family members rather than chemical imbalances or emotional disruptions that are often the focus of biomedical treatment approaches.

Second, the framework described here can be used instrumentally for clinical training in cultural competence, helping clinicians to reflect on potential clinician-client differences in how distress is conceptualized and on differences in preferences of healing and treatment. This will facilitate shared views on the problem, which is the foundation for treatment participation.

Third, the model described here may assist in intervention development globally by applying existing engagement practices or interventions in ways that consider the local cultural context. For example, although psychoeducation about services is acknowledged as a central practice utilized by clinicians to enhance engagement,[168] starting a discussion from the outset about psychotherapeutic services may be countercultural to ethnically diverse individuals' and families' conceptualization of distress (e.g., that the distress is a physical problem and not a mental health problem). A clinical psychologist in an outpatient setting told us about the complexities and challenges of engaging Hmong clients: "The Hmong did not engage depression care well in one of our clinics, but when the clinicians looked more closely (thanks to the Hmong LPN on staff), the Hmong didn't have a concept for depression. Once they taught the staff how to think in their terms of what we think of as depression, they engaged. Not rocket science, and yet it is" (Charles John Peek, e-mail communication, September 23, 2017).

Fourth, our chapter revealed that dovetailing engagement processes to the specific needs of Latino and Asian populations can be productive. One promising direction, for example, could be developing a menu of engagement interventions that are domain specific. This is an effective intervention approach that is utilized in child and family interventions.[169,170] Adapting interventions to address culturally specific concerns is another promising direction,[171,172] which has been demonstrated in ethnic-specific culturally adapted interventions.[173,174] The CIE can serve as a guiding framework for adapting evidence-based interventions for specific cultural groups by integrating adaptations within the multiple dimensions we have described in this chapter.

In conclusion, the chapter shows that a paradigm shift is urgently needed in conceptualizing mental health in engagement and treatment on a global level. It is critical to locate mental health and help-seeking ideas in the cultural context, respecting and acknowledging the variety of experiences of expressing mental health, mental distress, and healing and treatment, as well as the views of the people who help. To begin to understand the lived experiences of Latinos and Asians, Western concepts of mental health cannot be exported wholesale. Instead, having a shared understanding of various ways of expressing mental health and distress that integrates the nosology of Western and other cultural models of distress is necessary. An increased global awareness of diversity and the variation by which health and illness are expressed is essential for identifying and addressing the specific needs of ethnically diverse populations. To effectively address the mental health needs of the ethnically diverse individual requires understanding the person as a whole.

ACKNOWLEDGMENTS

This research was supported by a grant from the Agency of Healthcare Research and Quality to Dr. Yasui (AHRQ:5K12 HS023007). The authors thank Jonathan M. Storm for editorial support, Javier Escobar for thoughtful comments on the manuscript, and Zilin Cui for her assistance in the literature search.

REFERENCE LIST

1. World Health Organization. Mental Health Action Plan: 2013–2020. http://www .who.int/mental_health/publications/action_plan/en/www.who.int.
2. Wang PS, Lane M, Olfson M, et al. Twelve-month use of mental health services in the United States: Results from the National Comorbidity Survey Replication. *Archives of General Psychiatry.* 2005;62:629–640.
3. Addis ME, Wade WA, Hatgis C. Barriers to dissemination of evidence-based practices: Addressing practitioners' concerns about manual-based psychotherapies. *Clinical Psychology: Science and Practice.* 1999;6:430–441.
4. Chorpita BF, Yim LM, Donkervoet JC, et al. Toward large-scale implementation of empirically supported treatments for children: A review and observations by the Hawaii Empirical Basis to Services Task Force. *Clinical Psychology: Science and Practice.* 2002;9:165–190.
5. Hoagwood KE, Cavaleri MA, Olin SS, et al. Family support in children's mental health: a review and synthesis. *Clinical Child and Family Psychology Review.* 2010;13:1–45. doi:10.1007/s10567-009-0060-5.
6. McKay MM, Chasse KT, Paikoff R, et al. Family-level impact of the CHAMP Family Program: A community collaborative effort to support urban families and reduce youth HIV risk exposure. *Family Process.* 2004;43(1):79–93.
7. Alegria M, Green JG, McLaughlin KA, et al. *Disparities in Child and Adolescent Mental Health and Mental Health Services in the U.S.* New York: William T. Grant Foundation; 2015.
8. Johnson HC, Cournoyer DE, Fisher GA, et al. Children's emotional and behavioral disorders: Attributions of parental responsibility by professionals. *American Journal of Orthopsychiatry.* 2000;70(3):327–339.
9. McCabe KM. Factors that predict premature termination among Mexican-American children in outpatient psychotherapy. *Journal of Child and Family Studies.* 2002;11(3):347–359.
10. Stormshak EA, Dishion TJ, Light J, et al. Implementing family-centered interventions within the public middle school: Linking service delivery change to change in problem behavior. *Journal of Abnormal Child Psychology.* 2005;33:723–733.
11. Bernal GE, Domenech-Rodríguez MM. *Cultural Adaptations: Tools for Evidence-Based Practice with Diverse Populations.* American Psychological Association; 2012.
12. Betancourt H, Lopez SR. The study of culture, ethnicity, and race in American psychology. *American Psychologist.* 1993;48:629–637.
13. Alegría M, Pescosolido BA, Williams S, et al. Culture, race/ethnicity, and disparities: Fleshing out the socio-cultural framework for health services disparities. In: Rogers

A, McLeod J, Pescosolido BA, eds. *Handbook of the Sociology of Health, Illness, and Healing: A Blueprint for the 21st Century.* New York: Springer; 2011;363–382.

14. Cauce AM, Domenech-Rodríguez M, Paradise M, et al. Cultural and contextual influences in mental health help-seeking: A focus on ethnic minority youth. *Journal of Consulting and Clinical Psychology.* 2002;70(1):44–55.

15. Yasui M, Pottick KJ, Chen Y. Conceptualizing culturally infused engagement and its measurement for ethnic minority and immigrant children and families. *Clinical Child and Family Psychology Review.* 2017;20:250–332.

16. Kleinman A. Concepts and a model for the comparison of medical systems as cultural systems. *Social Science & Medicine.* 1978;12:85–93.

17. Ajzen I. The theory of planned behavior. *Organizational Behavior and Human Decision Processes.* 1991;50(2):79–211.

18. Gopalan G, Goldstein L, Klingenstein K. et al. Engaging families into child mental health treatment: Updates and special considerations. *Journal of the Canadian Academy of Child and Adolescent Psychiatry.* 2010;19(3):182–196.

19. McKay MM, Bannon Jr. WM. Engaging families in child mental health services. *Child and Adolescent Psychiatric Clinics of North America.* 2004;13(4):905–921.

20. Colby SL, Ortman JM. Projections of the size and composition of the U.S. population: 2014–2060. Current Population Reports. Washington, D.C.: U.S. Census Bureau; 2014:25–1143.

21. Derr AS. Mental health service use among immigrants in the United States: A systematic review. *Psychiatric Services.* 2016;67(3):265–274.

22. *Racial/Ethnic Differences in Mental Health Service Use among Adults.* HHS Publication No. SMA-15-4906. Rockville, Md.: Substance Abuse and Mental Health Services Administration; 2015.

23. Peters MD, Godfrey CM, Khalil H, et al. Guidance for conducting systematic scoping reviews. *International Journal of Evidence-Based Healthcare.* 2015;13:141–146.

24. Norris F. Epidemiology of trauma: Frequency and impact of different potentially traumatic events on different demographic groups. *Journal of Consulting and Clinical Psychology.* 1992;60:409–418.

25. Pole N, Gone JP, Kulkarni M. Posttraumatic stress disorder among ethnoracial minorities in the United States. *Clinical Psychology, Science and Practice.* 2008;15:35–61.

26. Ruef AM, Litz BT, Schlenger WE. Hispanic ethnicity and risk for combat-related posttraumatic stress disorder. *Cultural Diversity and Ethnic Minority Psychology.* 2000;6:235–251.

27. Contreras S, Fernandez S, Malcarne V, et al. Reliability and validity of the Beck depression and anxiety inventories in Caucasian Americans and Latinos. *Hispanic Journal of Behavioral Sciences.* 2004;26(4):446.

28. Beck AT, Steer RA, Carbin MG. Psychometric properties of the Beck Depression Inventory: Twenty-five years of evaluation. *Clinical Psychology Review.* 1988;8:77–100. doi:10.1016/.

29. Beck AT, Epstein N, Brown G, et al. An inventory for measuring clinical anxiety: Psychometric properties. *Journal of Consulting and Clinical Psychology.* 1988;56:893–897.

30. Crain R, Grzywacz JG, Schwantes M, et al. Correlates of mental health among Latino farmworkers in North Carolina. *Journal of Rural Health.* 2012;28(3):277–285. doi:10.1111/j.1748-0361.2011. 00401.x.

31. Kanel K. Mental health needs of Spanish-speaking Latinos in Southern California. *Hispanic Journal of Behavioral Services.* 2002;24:74–91.

32. Guarnaccia PJ. Ataques de Nervios in Puerto Rico: Culture Bound Syndrome or Popular Illness? *Medical Anthropology.* 1993;15:157–170.

33. Liebowitz MR, Salman E, Jusino C, et al. Ataque de Nervios and Panic Disorder. *American Journal of Psychiatry.* 1994;151(6):871–875.

34. Guarnaccia PJ, Martinez I, Acosta H. Mental health in the Hispanic immigrant community: An overview. In: Gonzales MJ, Gonzalez-Ramos G, eds. *Mental Health Care for New Hispanic Immigrants: Innovative Approaches in Contemporary Clinical Practice.* New York; 2005:161–189.

35. Guarnaccia PJ, Lewis-Fernandez R, Martinez I. Ataques de nervios as a marker of social and psychiatric vulnerability: Results from the NLAAS. *International Journal of Social Psychiatry.* 2010;56:289–309.

36. Keough ME, Timpano KR, Schmidt NB. Ataques de nervios: Culturally bound and distinct from panic attacks? *Depression and Anxiety.* 2009;26:16–21.

37. Lewis-Fernandez R, Gorritz M, Raggio GA, et al. Association of trauma-related disorders and dissociation with four idioms of distress among Latino psychiatric outpatients. *Culture, Medicine, and Psychiatry.* 2010;34:219–243.

38. Guarnaccia PJ, Lewis-Fernandez R, Marano MR. Toward a Puerto Rican popular nosology: Nervios and ataque de nervios. *Culture, Medicine, and Psychiatry.* 2003;27: 339–366.

39. Leon CA. El duende and other incubi: Suggestive interactions between culture and the brain. *Archives of General Psychiatry.* 1975;2:155–162.

40. Falicov CJ. Religion and spiritual folk traditions in immigrant families: Therapeutic resources with Latinos. In: Walsh F, ed. *Spiritual Resources in Family Therapy.* New York: Guilford Press;1999:104–120.

41. Bridges AJ, Andrews AR, Villalobos BT, et al. Does integrated behavioral health care reduce mental health disparities for Latinos? Initial findings. *Journal of Latina/o Psychology.* 2014;2:37–53.

42. Gerdes AC, Lawton KE, Haack LM, et al. Assessing ADHD in Latino Families: Evidence for Moving beyond Symptomatology. *Journal of Attention Disorders.* 2013;17:128–140.

43. Ornelas I, Perreira K. The Role of Migration in the Development of Depressive Symptoms among Immigrant Parents. *Social Science and Medicine.* 2011;73(8): 1169–1177.

44. Kessler RC, McGonagle K, Zhao S, et al. Lifetime and 12-month prevalence of DSM-III-R psychiatric disorders in the United States. *Archives of General Psychiatry.* 1994;51:8–19.

45. Zhang AY, Snowden LR. Ethnic characteristics of mental disorders in five U.S. communities. *Cultural Diversity and Ethnic Minority Psychology.* 1999;5:134–146.

46. Escobar JI, Randolph ET, Puente G, et al. Post-traumatic stress disorder in Hispanic Vietnam veterans: Clinical phenomenology and sociocultural characteristics. *Journal of Nervous and Mental Disease.* 1983;171:585–596.

47. Perilla JL, Norris FH, Lavizzo EA. Ethnicity, culture, and disaster response: Identifying and explaining ethnic differences in PTSD six months after Hurricane Andrew. *Journal of Social and Clinical Psychology.* 2002;21:20–45.

48. Bourque LB, Shen H. Psychometric characteristics of Spanish and English versions of the Civilian Mississippi Scale. *Journal of Traumatic Stress.* 2005;18(6):719–782.

49. De la Cancela V, Martinez IZ. An analysis of culturalism in Latino mental health: Folk medicine as a case in point. *Hispanic Journal of Behavioral Sciences.* 1983;5(3): 251–274.

50. Caplan S, Alvidrez J, Paris M, et al. Subjective versus objective: An exploratory analysis of Latino primary care patients with self-perceived depression who do not fulfill primary care evaluation of mental disorders patient health questionnaire criteria for depression. *The Primary Care Companion to the Journal of Clinical Psychiatry.* 2010;12, PCC.09m00899.

51. Viladrich A. From "shrinks" to "urban shamans": Argentine immigrants' therapeutic eclecticism in New York City. *Culture, Medicine, and Psychiatry.* 2007;3: 307–328.

52. Lewis-Fernandez R. Cultural Formulation of Psychiatric Diagnosis. *Culture, Medicine, and Psychiatry.* 1996;20:155–163.

53. Falicov CJ. Religion and spiritual traditions in immigrant families: Significance for Latino health and mental health. *Spiritual Resources in Family Therapy.* 2009;153–173.

54. Caplan S, Escobar J, Desai M, et al. Cultural influences upon causal beliefs about depression among Latino immigrants: Faith and resilience. *Journal of Transcultural Nursing.* 2013;24:68–77.

55. Cabassa LL, Hansen MC, Palinkas L, et al. Azucar y nervios: Explanatory models and treatment experiences of Hispanics with diabetes and depression. *Social Science and Medicine.* 2008;66:2413–2424.

56. Añez LM, Paris MJ, Bedregal LE, et al. Application of cultural constructs in the care of first-generation Latino clients in a community mental health setting. *Journal of Psychiatric Practice.* 2005;11:221–230.

57. Comas-Diaz L, Griffith EEH. *Clinical Guidelines in Cross-cultural Mental Health.* New York: Wiley; 1988.

58. Chapman MV, Stein GL. How do new immigrant Latino parents interpret problem behavior in adolescents? *Qualitative Social Work.* 2014;13(2):270–287.

59. Rogers A, Gallegos J. Pathways to health and mental health service utilization among older Mexicans and Mexican Americans. *International Social Work.* 2007;50(5): 654–670.

60. Kaltman S, De Mendoza AH, Gonzales FA. Preferences for trauma-related mental health services among Latina immigrants from Central America, South America, and Mexico. *Psychological Trauma: Theory, Research, Practice, and Policy.* 2014;6: 83–91.

61. Abdullah T, Brown TL. Mental illness stigma and ethnocultural beliefs, values, and norms: An integrative review. *Clinical Psychology Review*. 2011;31(6):934–948.

62. Cabassa LJ, Lester R, Zayas LH. It's like being in a labyrinth: Hispanic immigrants' perceptions of depression and attitudes toward treatments. *Journal of Immigrant and Minority Health*. 2007;9:1–16.

63. Applewhite SL. Curanderismo: Demystifying the health beliefs and practices of elderly Mexican Americans. *Health and Social Work*. 1995;20:247–253.

64. Unger JB, Ritt-Olson A, Teran L, et al. Cultural values and substance use in a multi-ethnic sample of California adolescents. *Addiction Research and Theory*. 2002;10: 257–279.

65. Interian A, Martinez IE, Guarnaccia PJ, et al. A qualitative analysis of the perception of stigma among Latinos receiving antidepressants. *Psychiatric Services*. 2007;58(12): 1591–1594.

66. Martinez Tyson D, Arriola N, Corvin J. Perceptions of depression and access to mental health care among Latino immigrants: Looking beyond one size. *Qualitative Health Research*. 2016;26(9):1289–1302.

67. Corrigan PW, Miller FE. Shame, blame, and contamination: A review of the impact of mental illness stigma on family members. *Journal of Mental Health*. 2004;13(6):537–548.

68. Corrigan PW, Penn DL. Lessons from social psychology on discrediting psychiatric stigma. *American Psychologist*. 1999;54(9):765–766.

69. Garcia CM, Gilchrist L, Vazquez G. Urban and rural immigrant Latino youths' and adults' knowledge and beliefs about mental health resources. *Journal of Immigrant and Minority Health*. 2011;13:500–509.

70. Frevert VS, Miranda AO, Kern RM. A conceptual formulation of the Latin culture and the treatment of Latinos from an Adlerian psychology perspective. *Journal of Individual Psychology*. 1998;54(3):292–309.

71. Luoma JB, Twohig MP, Waltz T. An investigation of stigma in individuals receiving treatment for substance abuse. *Addictive Behaviors*. 2007;32:1331–1346.

72. Kouyoumdjian H, Zamboanga BL, Hansen DJ. Barriers to mental health services for Latinos: Treatment and research considerations. *Clinical Psychology: Science and Practice*. 2003;10:394–422. doi:10.1093/clipsy.bpg041.

73. Rothe EM. Considering cultural diversity in the management of ADHD in Hispanic patients. Supplement to the *Journal of the National Medical Association*. 2005;97:17S–23S.

74. Altarriba J, Bauer LM. Counseling the Hispanic client: Cuban Americans, Mexican Americans, and Puerto Ricans. *Journal of Counseling and Development*. 1998;76:389–396.

75. Cuéllar I, Arnold B, González G. Cognitive referents of acculturation: Assessment of cultural constructs in Mexican Americans. *Journal of Community Psychology*. 1995;2: 339–355.

76. Sorenson SB, Siegel JM. Gender, ethnicity, and sexual assault: Findings from a Los Angeles study. *Journal of Social Issues*. 1992;48:93–104.

77. Ishikawa RZ, Cardemil EV, Falmagne RJ. Help seeking and help receiving for emotional distress among Latino men and women. *Qualitative Health Research*. 2010;20: 1558–1572. doi:10.1177/1049732310369140.

78. Magaña SM, Ramírez García JI, Hernández MG, et al. Psychological distress among Latino family caregivers of adults with schizophrenia: The roles of burden and stigma. *Psychiatric Services*. 2007;58:378–384. doi:10.1176/appi.ps.58.3.378.

79. Marquez JA, Ramirez Garcia JI. Family caregivers' narratives of mental health treatment usage processes by their Latino adult relatives with serious and persistent mental illness. *Journal of Family Psychology*. 2013;27:398–408.

80. Arcaya J. Hispanic American boys and adolescent males. In: Horne AM, Kiselica MS, eds. *Handbook of Counseling Boys and Adolescent Males: A Practitioners' Guide*. Thousand Oaks, Calif.: Sage Publications; 1999:101–116.

81. Garcia-Preto N. Latino families: An overview. In: McGoldrick M, Giordano J, Pearce JK, eds. *Ethnicity and Family Therapy*. New York: Guilford Press; 1996:141–154.

82. Zea MC, Mason MA, Murguia A. Latino/Latina religious traditions: Implications for psychotherapy. In: Bergin AE, Richards PS, eds. *Psychotherapy and Religious Diversity: A Guide for Mental Health Professionals*. Washington, D.C.: American Psychological Association; 2000:397–419.

83. Fraga ED, Atkinson DR, Wampold BE. Ethnic group preferences for multicultural counseling competencies. *Cultural Diversity and Ethnic Minority Psychology*. 2004;10(1): 53–65. doi:10.1037/1099-9809.10.1.53.

84. Ortega AN, Alegría M. Self-reliance, mental health need, and the use of mental healthcare among island Puerto Ricans. *Mental Health Services Research*, 2002;4(3): 131–140.

85. Alegria M, Mulvaney-Day N, Torres M. Prevalence of psychiatric disorders across Latino subgroups in the United States. *American Journal of Public Health*. 2007;97: 68–75.

86. Vega WA, Alegria M. Latino mental health and treatment. In: Aguirre-Molina M, Molina C, Zambrana R, eds. *Latino Health in the United States*. New York: Jossey-Bass 2001.

87. Arredondo P, Perez P. Expanding multicultural competence through social justice leadership. *Counseling Psychologist*. 2003;31(3):282–289.

88. Gil RM, Vasquez CI. *The Maria Paradox*. New York: G. P. Putnam; 1996.

89. Ginorio AB, Gutierrez L, Cauce AM. Psychological issues for Latinas. In: Landrine H., ed. *Bringing Cultural Diversity to Feminist Psychology*. Washington, D.C.: American Psychological Association; 1995:241–263.

90. Weisman A. Integrating culturally based approaches with existing interventions for Hispanic/Latino families coping with schizophrenia. *Psychotherapy: Theory, Research, Practice, Training*. 2005;41:178–197.

91. Mann A, Garcia A. Characteristics of community interventions to decrease depression in Mexican American women. *Hispanic Health Care International*. 2005;3: 87–93.

92. Mendelson C. Health perceptions of Mexican American women. *Journal of Transcultural Nursing.* 2002;13:210–217.

93. Brandon G. The uses of plants in healing in an Afro-Cuba religion: Santeria. *Journal of Black Studies.* 1991;22:51–76.

94. Rojas-Vilches AP, Negy C, Reig Ferrer A. Attitudes toward seeking therapy among Puerto Rican and Cuban American young adults and their parents. *International Journal of Clinical and Health Psychology.* 2011;11:313–341.

95. Jenkins, JH. *Extraordinary Conditions: Culture and Experience in Mental Illness.* Oakland: University of California Press; 2015.

96. Miville M, Constantine M. Sociocultural predictors of psychological help-seeking attitudes and behavior among Mexican American college students. *Peace Research Abstracts Journal.* 2007;44(3):420.

97. Arcia E, Fernandez MC, Jaquez M. Latina mothers' stances on stimulant medication: Complexity, conflict, and compromise. *Developmental and Behavioral Pediatrics.* 2004;25: 311–317.

98. Kaltman S, Green BL, Mete M, et al. Trauma, depression, and comorbid PTSD/depression in a community sample of Latina immigrants. *Psychological Trauma: Theory, Research Practice, and Policy.* 2010;2:31–39. doi:10.1037/a0018952.

99. Parra-Cardona JR, DeAndrea DC. Latinos' access to online and formal mental health support. *Journal of Behavioral Health Services and Research.* 2016;43:281–292.

100. Centers for Disease Control and Prevention. *Health, United States, 2012, with Special Feature on Emergency Care.* https://www.cdc.gov/nchs/data/hus/hus12.pdf.

101. Escarce JJ, Kapur K. Access to a quality of healthcare. In: Tienda M, Mitchell F, eds. *National Research Council: Hispanics and the Future of America.* Washington, D.C.: National Academies Press; 2006;410–446.

102. Sadler GR, Ryujin L, Nguyen T. Heterogeneity within the Asian American community. *International Journal for Equity in Health.* 2004;2:12.

103. U.S. Census Bureau, 2012. *The Asian Population: 2010.* http://www.census.gov/library/publications/2012/dec/c2010br-11.html.

104. Chou C, Tulolo A, Raver EW, et al. Effect of race and health insurance on health disparities: Results from the National Health Interview Survey. *Journal of Health Care for the Poor and Underserved.* 2013;24:1353–1363.

105. Andrew G, Cohen A, Salgaonkar S, et al. The explanatory models of depression and anxiety in primary care: A qualitative study from India. *BMC Research Notes.* 2012;5:499.

106. Hsiao FH, Klimidis S, Minas HI, et al. Folk concepts of mental disorders among Chinese- Australian patients and their caregivers. *Journal of Advanced Nursing.* 2006;55: 58–67.

107. Muecke MA. In search of healers: Southeast Asian refugees in the American health care system. *Western Journal of Medicine.* 1983;139:835–840.

108. Choi KH. Psychological separation-individuation and adjustment to college among Korean American students: The roles of collectivism and individualism. *Journal of Counseling Psychology.* 2002;49(4):468–475.

109. Bazzoui W. Affective disorders in Iraq. *British Journal of Psychiatry*. 1970;117:195–203. DOI: https://doi.org/10.1192/S0007125000192888

110. Kumar A, Nevid JS. Acculturation, enculturation, and perceptions of mental disorders in Asian Indian immigrants. *Cultural Diversity and Ethnic Minority Psychology*. 2010;16:274–283.

111. Ying YW. Explanatory models of major depression and implications for help-seeking among immigrant Chinese-American women. *Culture, Medicine, Psychiatry*. 1990;14:393–405.

112. Lin KM. Traditional Chinese medical beliefs and their relevance for mental illness and psychiatry. In: Kleinman A, Lin TY, eds. *Normal and Abnormal Behavior in Chinese Culture*. Boston: D. Reidel; 1980:95–111.

113. *Diagnostic and Statistical Manual of Mental Disorders-IV*. Washington D.C.: American Psychiatric Association; 1994.

114. Pang KYC. Hwabyung: The construction of a Korean popular illness among Korean elderly immigrant women in the United States. *Cultural Medical Psychiatry*. 1990;14:495–512.

115. Al-Krenawi A. Family therapy with a multiparental/multispousal family. *Family Process*. 1998;37(1):65–82.

116. D'Avanzo CE, Barab SA. Depression and anxiety among Cambodian refugee women in France and the United States. *Mental Health Nursing*. 1998;19:541–556.

117. Marsella A, Kinzie D, Gordon P. Ethnic variations in the expression of depression. *Journal of Cross-Cultural Psychology*. 1973;4:435–458.

118. Hwang W, Myers HF, Abe-Kim J, et al. A conceptual paradigm for understanding culture's impact on mental health: The Cultural Influences on Mental Health (CIMH) Model. *Clinical Psychology Review*. 2008;28:212–228.

119. Liu D, Hinton L, Tran C, et al. Reexamining the relationships among dementia, stigma, and aging in immigrant Chinese and Vietnamese family caregivers. *Journal of Cross-cultural Gerontology*. 2008;23:289–299.

120. Anand A, Cochrane R. The mental health status of South Asian women in Britain: A review of the U.K. literature. *Psychology and Developing Societies*. 2005;17:195–214.

121. Frye BA, McGill D. Cambodian refugee adolescents: Cultural factors and mental health nursing. *Journal of Child and Adolescent Psychiatric Nursing*. 1993;6:24–31.

122. Yeung A, Chang D, Gresham Jr. RL, et al. Illness beliefs of depressed Chinese American patients in primary care. *Journal of Nervous and Mental Disease*. 2004;192(4): 324–327.

123. Shyu Y, Tsai J, Tsai W. Explaining and selecting treatments for autism: Parental explanatory models in Taiwan. *Journal of Autism and Developmental Disorders*. 2010; 40:1323–1331. doi:10.1007/s10803-010-0991-1.

124. Al-Krenawi A, Graham JR, Maoz B. The healing significance of the Negev's Bedouin Dervish. *Social Science and Medicine*. 1996;43:13–21.

125. Daie N, Witztum E, Mark M, et al. The belief in the transmigration of souls: Psychotherapy of a Druze patient with severe anxiety reaction. *British Journal of Medical Psychology*. 1992;65:119–130.

126. Somasundaram DJ, van de Put WACM, Eisenbruch M, et al. Starting mental health services in Cambodia. *Social Science and Medicine*. 1999;48:1029–1046.

127. Mathews M. Assessment and comparison of culturally based explanations for mental disorder among Singaporean Chinese youth. *International Journal of Social Psychiatry*. 2011;57(1):3–17.

128. Al-Krenawi A, Graham JR. Culturally sensitive social work practice with Arab clients in mental health settings. *Health and Social Work*. 2000;25:9–22.

129. Lee S, Juon HS, Martinez G, et al. Model minority at risk: Expressed needs of mental health by Asian American young adults. *Journal of Community Health*. 2009;34:144–152.

130. Hsiao FH, Klimidis S, Minas H, et al. Cultural attribution of mental health suffering in Chinese societies: The views of Chinese patients with mental illness and their caregivers. *Journal of Clinical Nursing*. 2005;15:998–1006.

131. Caplan N, Choy MH, Whitmore JK. *Children of the Boat People: A Study of Educational Success*. Ann Arbor: University of Michigan Press; 1991.

132. Zhou M, Bankston III CL. *Growing Up American: The Adaptation of Vietnamese Adolescents in the United States*. New York: Russell Sage Foundation; 1998.

133. Phillips MR, Li Y, Stroup TS, et al. Causes of schizophrenia reported by patients' family members in China. *British Journal of Psychiatry*. 2000;177:20–25.

134. Yang L, Philips MR, Lo G, et al. "Excessive thinking" as explanatory model for schizophrenia: Impacts on stigma and moral status in mainland China. *Schizophrenia Bulletin*. 2010;36:836–845.

135. Park YJ, Ryu H, Han KS, et al. Anger, anger expression, and suicidal ideation in Korean adolescents. *Archives of Psychiatric Nursing*. 2010;24:168–177.

136. Yong F, McCallion P. Hwabyung as caregiving stress among Korean-American caregivers of a relative with dementia. *Journal of Gerontological Social Work*. 2004;42(2): 3–19.

137. Guzder J, Krishna M. Sita-Shakti: Cultural paradigms for Indian women. *Transcultural Psychiatric Research Review*. 1991;28(4):257–301.

138. Ng CH. The stigma of mental illness in Asian cultures. *Australian and New Zealand Journal of Psychiatry*. 1997;31:382–390.

139. Yang LH, Phelan JC, Link BG. Stigma and beliefs of efficacy towards traditional Chinese medicine and Western psychiatric treatment among Chinese-Americans. *Cultural Diversity and Ethnic Minority Psychology*. 2008;14(1):10–18.

140. Sun B, Fan N, Zhang M, et al. Attitudes towards people with mental illness among psychiatrists, psychiatric nurses, involved family members, and the general population in a large city in Guangzhou, China. *International Journal of Mental Health Systems*. 2014;8:26.

141. Mak WWS. Integrative model of caregiving: How macro and micro factors affect caregivers of adults with severe and persistent mental illness. *American Journal of Orthopsychiatry*. 2005;75(1):40–53.

142. Mak WWS, Cheung RYM. Affiliate stigma among caregivers of people with intellectual disability or mental illness. *Journal of Applied Research in Intellectual Disabilities*, 2008;21:532–545.

143. Mak WWS, Cheung RYM. Psychological distress and subjective burden of caregivers of people with mental illness: The role of affiliate stigma and face concern. *Community Mental Health Journal*. 2012;48(3):270–274.

144. Singh I. Doing their jobs: Mothering with Ritalin in a culture of mother-blame. *Social Science and Medicine*. 2004;59(6):1193–1205.

145. Savaya R. The under-use of psychological services by Israeli Arabs: An examination of the roles of negative attitudes and the use of alternative sources of help. *International Social Work*. 1998;41:195–209.

146. Kim MT. Measuring depression in Korean Americans: Development of the Kim depression scale for Korean Americans. *Journal of Transcultural Nursing*. 2002;13:109–117.

147. Yeh C, Inose M. Difficulties and coping strategies of Chinese, Japanese, and Korean immigrant students. *Adolescence*. 2002;37:69–82.

148. Yasui M. Cultural dimensions of mental health and approaches to treatment: A dual approach in the exploratory examination of mental health beliefs, practices, and experiences of Chinese American and immigrant youth and families. In: Choi Y, Hahm HC, eds. *Asian American Parenting: Family Process and Intervention*. New York: Springer; 2017:193–208.

149. Cheung FM. Conceptualization of psychiatric illness and help-seeking behavior among Chinese. *Culture, Medicine, and Psychiatry*. 1987;11:97–106.

150. Park SY, Bernstein KS. Depression and Korean American immigrants. *Archives of Psychiatric Nursing*. 2002;22:12–19.

151. Akutsu PD, Castillo ED, Snowden LR. Differential referral patterns to ethnic-specific and mainstream mental health programs for four Asian American groups. *American Journal of Orthopsychiatry*. 2007;77:95–103.

152. Ahmad I, Macaskill A, Tabassum R. Attitudes towards mental health in an urban Pakistani community in the United Kingdom. *International Journal of Social Psychiatry*. 2000;46(3):170–181.

153. Atkinson DR, Ponterotto JG, Sanchez AR. Attitudes of Vietnamese and Anglo-American students toward counseling. *Journal of College Student Personnel*. 1984;25:448–452.

154. Leong FTL, Lau ASL. Barriers to providing effective mental health services to Asian Americans. *Mental Health Services Research*. 2001;3(4):201–214.

155. Sue DW, Sue D. *Counseling the Culturally Diverse: Theory and Practice*. New York: John Wiley & Sons; 2003.

156. Sheikh S, Furnham A. A cross-cultural study of mental health beliefs and attitudes towards seeking professional help. *Social Psychiatry and Psychiatric Epidemiology*. 2000;35:326–334.

157. Fung K, Wong YLR. Factors influencing attitudes towards seeking professional help among East and Southeast Asian immigrant and refugee women. *International Journal of Social Psychiatry*. 2007;53:216–231.

158. Cheung FM, Lee S, Chan Y. Variations in problem conceptualizations and intended solutions among Hong Kong students. *Culture, Medicine, and Psychiatry*. 1983;7(3):263–278.

159. Kim BSK. Adherence to Asian and European American cultural values and attitudes toward seeking professional psychological help among Asian American college students. *Journal of Counseling Psychology.* 2007;54:474–480.

160. Fan C. A comparison of attitudes towards mental illness and knowledge of mental health services between Australian and Asian students. *Community Mental Health Journal.* 1999;35(1):47–56.

161. Tran UNTL. Vietnamese immigrants in Brisbane, Australia: Perception of parenting roles, child development, child health, illness, and disability, and health service utilisation. *International Journal of Population Research.* 2012. Article ID 932364. doi: 10.1155/2012/932364.

162. Abe-Kim J, Takeuchi DT, Hwang WC. Predictors of help-seeking for emotional distress among Chinese Americans: Family matters. *Journal of Consulting and Clinical Psychology.* 2002;70(5):1186–1190.

163. Chin D, Takeuchi DT, Suh D. Access to health care among Chinese, Korean, and Vietnamese Americans. In: Hogue C, Hargraves MA, Collins KS, eds. *Minority Health in America.* Baltimore: Johns Hopkins University Press; 2000:77–98.

164. Wong EC, Marshall GN, Schell TL, et al. Barriers to mental health care utilization for U.S. Cambodian refugees. *Journal of Consulting and Clinical Psychology.* 2006;74:1116–1120.

165. Bernal G, Bonilla J, Bellido C. Ecological validity and cultural sensitivity for outcome research: Issues for the cultural adaptation and development of psychosocial treatments with Hispanics. *Journal of Abnormal Child Psychology.* 1995;23(1):67–82.

166. New Freedom Commission. *Achieving the Promise: Transforming Mental Health Care in America.* Final report (Pub No. SMA-03-3832). Bethesda, Md.: U.S. Department of Health and Human Services; 2003.

167. Sue S. In search of cultural competence in psychotherapy and counseling. *American Psychologist.* 1998;53:440–448.

168. Becker KD, Lee BR, Daleiden EL, et al. The common elements of engagement in children's mental health services: Which elements for which outcomes? *Journal of Clinical Child and Adolescent Psychology.* 2015;44(1):30–43.

169. Webster-Stratton C. A randomized trial of two parent training programs for families with conduct-disordered children. *Journal of Consulting and Clinical Psychology.* 1984;52(4):666–678.

170. Dishion TJ, Stormshak EA. *Intervening in Children's Lives: An Ecological, Family-Centered Approach to Mental Health Care.* Washington, D.C.: American Psychological Association; 2007.

171. Barrera Jr. M, Castro FG. A heuristic framework for the cultural adaptation of interventions. *Clinical Psychology: Science and Practice.* 2006;13(4):311–316.

172. Comas-Díaz L. Cultural variation in the therapeutic relationship. In: Goodheart, CD, Kazdin, AE, Sternberg, RJ. *Evidence-Based Psychotherapy: Where Practice and Research Meet.* Washington, D.C.: American Psychological Association; 2006:81–105.

173. Miranda J, Azocar F, Organista K, Dwyer E, Arean P. Treatment of depression among impoverished primary care patients from ethnic minority groups disadvantaged medical patients. *Psychiatric Services.* 2003;54(2):219–225.

174. Miranda, J, Schoenbaum M, Sherbourne C, Duan N, Wells, K. The effects of primary care depression treatment on minority patients' clinical status and employment. *Archives of General Psychiatry.* 2004;61(8):827–834.

3 · THE ABUSE OF PSYCHIATRY GLOBALLY

A Focus on a Little-Known Historical Example from Francoist Spain

ETHAN PEARLSTEIN AND JAVIER I. ESCOBAR

INTRODUCTION

Given the cost of and the burden imposed by mental disorders globally, and in particular, the lack of equity across world regions related to services and attention paid to mental disorders, there is a need to implement, adapt, and expand specialized mental health programs, particularly in low and middle-income countries. While most of these influences are expected to be positive, the unrestrained expansion and the growing influence of psychiatry globally may also have the potential of using psychiatry as a tool for political purposes, particularly when it becomes an instrument of the state.

In this chapter, we present some historical examples of how the specialty of psychiatry, including its academic branches, has been used in the past for political purposes, particularly by totalitarian states. These examples illustrate some specific instances of the use of psychiatric labels or interventions in efforts to justify the detention, silencing, and ostracizing of political dissenters. This retrospective look at historical events provides support to the notion that often times psychiatry has been used to deal with political deviance or disobedience through the labeling of certain behaviors or attitudes as "mental disorders." This long and painful global history should elicit warnings and caveats on the potential negative influences and untoward consequences of psychiatric theory and practice. Our primary focus will be on Spain during the Franco years, presenting a little-known example of the abuse of psychiatry and the psychiatric labeling of enemies of the regime.

Clearly, psychiatry has been a more common instrument of abuse than other medical specialties. The use of psychiatric labeling as a political tool has been facilitated by the subjective nature of the clinical presentations, the lack of objective or reliable diagnostic markers, the emphasis on observed or reported "behaviors," and the stigma surrounding mental disorders.

As part of a review of the best-documented global instances of institutional abuse of medicine and psychiatry, we will highlight five other examples before addressing the Francoist regime.

Nazi Germany, 1938–1941

The tragic isolation and mass murder of the "physically and mentally unfit" as part of the "euthanasia" program termed Aktion T-4 saw the deaths of at least 71,088 persons, many at the hands of leading academic psychiatrists.[1] The Aktion T-4 program began in September 1939 with a brief and inconspicuous note from Adolf Hitler authorizing psychiatrists with the "responsibility to extend doctors' powers in such a way that after most careful assessment of their condition, those suffering from illness deemed to be incurable may be granted a mercy death." The project began first in 1939 with the killing of over 5,200 children with suspected mental and physical illness, and the murder of thousands of Polish psychiatric patients to provide barrack space for German soldiers.[2] Later the operation became well organized, with a central office at Tiergartenstrasse Nr. 4 in Berlin, hence the name of the project, Aktion T-4, and a front organization named the Reich Committee for the Scientific Registration of Serious Hereditary-and Congenitally-based Illnesses. Using grey postal vans so as to appear inconspicuous, a transport service would collect patients and transfer them to one of six asylums (Grafeneck, Brandenburg, Hartheim, Pirna-Sonnenstein, Bernburg, or Hadamar), where they were murdered. Form letters were sent to families informing them first of a transfer to a new asylum, and then a letter of condolence explaining that their loved one had died, generally from a rapidly fatal and terminal disease.[2]

The project continued for four years under the direction of Karl Brandt, Hitler's personal physician and professor of psychiatry at Würzburg University, and it exceeded its global target of 70,000 deaths. The genocide came into the public sphere after a notable protest in August 1941 by Clemens August, Count von Galen, Bishop of Münster, who in a strongly worded sermon stated, "It is only necessary for some secret edict to order that the method developed for the mentally ill should be extended to other 'unproductive' people.... Then none of our lives will be safe anymore." Hitler issued a halt order on August 24, 1941, which put an end to the mass gassing of psychiatric patients specifically but did not stop euthanasia practices in Nazi Germany. In fact, technological advances developed during the Aktion T-4 program, such as the use of lethal gases for the mass murder of innocent civilians, were continued. The same gas chambers from the asylums would later be used for concentration camp prisoners, forced laborers, children residing in orphanages, and countless others.[2]

The Soviet Union during the 1960s

In the old Soviet Union, examples of the abuse of psychiatry included the forced isolation and treatment of political dissenters in mental hospitals and the use of highly questionable diagnostic labels such as "sluggish schizophrenia." These strategies were used for the purpose of discrediting those who held beliefs or behaviors that were contrary to those of the Soviet regime.[2] Thus, the use of psychiatry by the state played a central role in the socialist government of the Soviet Union, with those who opposed the creation of an idealistic and restrictive society being classified, by default, as mentally ill. Unlike other medical specialties, psychiatry played the unique role of depriving many individuals who had been labeled as mentally ill of their civil liberties, in the name of protecting a perfect society.

The diagnosis of "sluggish schizophrenia" was based upon the work of Andrei Snezhnevsky, the director of the Institute of Psychiatry of the USSR Academy of Medical Sciences. The rationale was terribly simple. It assumed that since there would be no logical reason for an individual to oppose such a perfect system as communism, there had to be something terribly wrong, and therefore a medical (psychiatric) diagnosis had to be applied to such an individual. The diagnostic criteria and the clinical terms often used also included "antisocial behavior," "anxiety," "poor social adaptation," "unrealistic ideas" (e.g., about reforming society), "strong religious convictions," and "confrontation and defiance of the authorities."

A key element for many of these psychiatric diagnoses was "the capacity to behave normally for considerable periods," thereby allowing the diagnosis to be made even in the case of people who currently showed no overt signs of mental illness.[3]

By April 1969, Yuri Andropov, head of the Committee for State Security (the KGB), had begun work on establishing a network of mental asylums for the purpose of defending the Soviet government from the "mentally infirm" dissenters. This system allowed psychiatrists to create specific diagnoses for political dissenters and to justify the detention of political dissidents without court proceedings.[3]

In January 1971, Soviet psychiatrist Semyon Gluzman published a report articulating that political dissidence could not be equated with mental illness. For doing this, Gluzman was sentenced to seven years of imprisonment. This act, however, brought some national and international attention to this issue and ignited further activism and inquiries into the actions of the Soviet government and the imprisonment of political dissidents. This would lead eventually to the resignation of the USSR's All-Union Society of Neurologists and Psychiatrists from the World Psychiatric Association in 1983.[3] The American Psychiatric Association in the United States had become aware of many of these abuses, and for many years several members of APA committees traveled to the USSR and produced several reports documenting them.

The People's Republic of China under Mao Zedong

During the dictatorship of Mao Zedong, Chinese authorities viewed what may have been simply peaceful demonstrations of political protest as serious manifestations of psychiatric problems. Many of the individuals who demonstrated were imprisoned for long periods of time, often receiving such psychiatric diagnoses as "paranoid psychosis," despite the lack of any medical evidence for the validity of these diagnoses.[4]

The abuse of psychiatry for the detention of political dissidents reached its peak in China during the Cultural Revolution, between 1966 and 1976, also under Mao's leadership. In building its communist regime, China relied heavily on the experiences and support of the Soviet Union, which provided scientific and technological assistance to the Chinese government. Thus, the new generation of psychiatric professionals that emerged in China after 1949 was overwhelmingly influenced by Soviet psychiatric theory and doctrine.[5]

One area of mental health theory and practice that was particularly appealing to the Chinese political regime was forensic psychiatry, a field that came to be widely employed for the purpose of equating political and religious dissent with mental illness. Apart from forensic psychiatry, the field of psychiatry in general fared rather poorly from a global perspective. Under the leadership of Mao, mental health institutions were dismantled entirely throughout the country, and many psychiatric professionals were forcibly removed from their positions and labeled as "bourgeois academic authorities."[5] Also, due to Mao's reductionist philosophy, political adherence was the key to social survival and good mental health; therefore, the appropriate treatment for mental illness was further political education and imprisonment.[5]

As was the case with the Soviet Union, the Chinese employed political psychiatry as a repressive measure. Detainees were brutally beaten and subjected to medical treatment, largely as a form of punishment. Thus, in the middle of the twentieth century, psychiatric medicine in China was quite limited in its reach, particularly regarding the use of effective and modern interventions for managing mental disorders.

Several drastic interventions emerging in Europe during the early ages of scientific psychiatry—including insulin coma therapy (Manfred Sakel, a Polish psychiatrist in 1927), electroconvulsive therapy, or ECT (Ugo Cerletti and Lucio Bini, Italian neurologists in 1937), and prefrontal lobotomy (Egas Moniz, a Portuguese neuropsychiatrist in 1936)—were largely discarded and discouraged (except ECT) from the therapeutic armamentarium of most countries by the early 1950s, following the arrival of new and effective pharmacological treatments such as chlorpromazine and other antipsychotic medications. However, the use of these old interventions continued in China, with many reports on the use of prefrontal lobotomy, the widespread use of ECT, and insulin coma therapy into the late 1950s. It is suspected that these interventions may have been used on political dissenters as a form of punishment.[5]

More recently, a religious sect known as the Falun Gong became the target of forced imprisonment and forensic psychiatric analysis. In response to mounting criticism of their movement, in April 1999 the group held the largest public demonstration in China since the Tiananmen protests of May 1989, a daylong silent protest of over 10,000 people. Suddenly, nearly two months later, dozens of high-ranking officials in the group were arrested and detained in the middle of the night. Since then, thousands of practitioners have been similarly arrested and detained; several reports indicate that as many as seventy followers have died as a result of their imprisonment.[5] It has been reported that in mental asylums throughout the country, many Falun Gong practitioners may be subjected to forceful psychiatric interventions, including psychiatric drugs, frequent use of restraints and isolation, treatment with ECT, and electrical acupuncture treatment. They may even be forced to "convert," through renouncing their belief in the Falun Gong sect, as a precondition for their eventual release.[5] While we cannot be certain of the validity of these reports, as we do not have the official perspective of reliable psychiatry sources in China or documentation on whether or not some Falun Gong practitioners were truly mentally ill, this should raise awareness that the potential for psychiatric abuse is always present around the globe.

Cuba, 1940s and 1950s

Prior to the Cuban Revolution, prominent physician-eugenicists such as José Chelala Aguilera and Angel C. Arce published and lectured widely on "sexual hetero-normativity" around the time of the Second Cuban Republic (1933–1950), with the goal of educating the public on the dangers of deviating from "traditional" family dynamics and resorting to divorce and juvenile delinquency.

This approach seems to be quite different from the state-sponsored abuses of psychiatry that have been mentioned earlier, as it was primarily a moralistic initiative whose target was the education of the Cuban layperson via accessible media outlets, such as periodicals, newspapers, and radio shows.[6]

José Chelala Aguilera (1906–1987), a central figure in Cuban eugenics, was a practicing obstetrician and gynecologist in Havana as well as a professor of medicine at the University of Havana. By the 1940s, Chelala became a household name in Cuba for his widely read column "Problemas de medicina social" (Problems of social medicine) published in *Bohemia*, a popular Cuban variety magazine. To Chelala, the country's rising divorce rate was a major problem that needed to be addressed through public education, with an emphasis on the importance of sexual health and the stability of marriage and the family unit.[6]

Angel Arce (1892–1967), also a physician and prominent Cuban eugenicist, believed that engaging the public in formal sexual education programs would put an end to the "hereditary and contagious damage" of the future offspring.[7] Like Chelala, Arce utilized various media outlets to spread his message, including national newspaper and radio. Arce was perhaps best known, however, for his Institute of Sexology in Havana, as well as its monthly magazine, *Sexología: Mensuario revista paramédica* (Sexology: Monthly popular medical magazine). The magazine was published and distributed widely throughout Cuba and included sections in which Arce would respond to questions from the Cuban public. At his institute, Arce offered sexual education courses, including some aimed at working Cubans and some offered on weekends.[6] (We will see elements of these "moral concerns" also in the example from Spain to be presented below.)

Physicians such as Arce and Chelala saw it as their duty to educate the public in part because of the failure of the Cuban government to enact eugenics legislation. A law that would have required couples to undergo mandatory prenuptial medical examination and health certification was introduced in 1940 and launched a fierce medical debate on both sides. Chelala, on the radio program *Universidad del aire* (University on the air), remarked that this health "certificate is a miniscule fragment, almost microscopic, of a sweeping social-medicine project adapted to Cuba and the particular conditions of Cuba that we [medical professionals] have been presenting . . . for years."[6] The law ultimately failed to pass, but the effort to get this legislation through, serves as a demonstration of the increased focus placed by these academics on imposing an eugenic theory upon the Cuban layperson independent from the government.

The United States of America

The United States also has well-documented historical instances of the abuse of medicine and psychiatry, especially as it relates to the mistreatment of African Americans. The Tuskegee experiment, an infamous syphilis study carried out in Macon County, Alabama, between 1932 and 1972, still resonates today as a glaring example of medical abuse imposed on an ethnic minority.

Slavery and mental health. Regarding psychiatric abuse, a viewpoint commonly expressed by American psychiatrists mainly from Southern states in the nineteenth century—based upon data of admission to asylums throughout the United States—was that enslavement may be protective to the mental health of African Americans. By contrast, freedom from enslavement, as evidenced in the Northern states, was theorized to predispose freed slaves to mental illness.[8]

Thus, in this instance, the psychiatric community, affected by bias reinforced by suspicious hospital statistics, incorporated the notion that the freed slave may constitute a threat to American society, thus creating new diagnoses specifically for this purpose.[9]

In May 1851, American physician Samuel Cartwright, then chairman of the Louisiana Medical Association, published an essay titled "Report on the Diseases and Physical Peculiarities of the Negro Race." In his work, Cartwright contends that African Americans are inferior by comparison to whites and identifies two new mental illnesses affecting them: "drapetomania," or the escape of a slave from a white master, and "dysaesthesia aethiopis," characterized by the slave neglecting or refusing to work.[10] Cartwright states that to prevent the enslaved from running away, they should be adequately fed and clothed and allowed to keep a fire at night. When such measures are taken and slaves are still inclined to escape, however, "they should be punished until they fall into that submissive state which it was intended for them to occupy."[10] In describing the disease of "dysaesthesia aeithiopis," Cartwright draws upon the Declaration of Independence to lend credence to his argument. He writes that the document "was drawn up at a time when negroes were scarcely considered as human beings," and that the sentence "*all men are by nature free and equal*" was only intended to apply to white men, emphasizing "the false dogma that all mankind possesses the same mental, physiological and anatomical organization, and that the liberty, free institutions, and whatever else would be a blessing to one portion, would, under the same external circumstances, be to all, without regard to any original or internal differences inherent in the organization."[10] In Cartwright's opinion, while life, liberty, and the pursuit of happiness should be encouraged in whites, the same cannot be said of African Americans, who should be enslaved for their own mental health. This medicalization of black protest played centrally into the perpetuation of slavery in the United States.[8]

Homosexuality as mental disorder. It must also be noted that homosexuality was an official psychiatric diagnosis in North America and that it officially appeared in the first two editions of the *Diagnostic and Statistical Manual of Mental Disorders* of the American Psychiatric Association (DSM-I, DSM-II) under the category of "sexual deviations."

While the diagnosis was formally removed from the manual in 1973 following a vote of the APA membership, the DSM-III published in 1980 and the DSM-III R published in 1987 continued to include the label "homo-sexuality," this time characterized as "ego-dystonic homosexuality."

It is of interest to point out that in some countries, such as Chile, "homo-sexuality" was apparently the target of governmental actions. As history tells it, the dictator Carlos Ibáñez del Campo arrested and raided places frequented by homosexuals up to the 1950s and passed law no. 11625 on *estados antisociales and medidas de seguridad* (antisocial conditions and security measures), which included homosexuality. An unverifiable legend adds that these prisoners were placed in boats and that those boats were sunk into the ocean with the prisoners inside, an action called *fondeamiento*.

Misdiagnosis of psychosis in African Americans. Another unfortunate example of misdiagnoses that is well documented in the scientific literature is that of African American patients suffering from major psychoses and schizophrenia in numbers greater than those of other ethnic groups. This "diagnostic bias" seems related to "information and criterion variance."[11,12] A similar misdiagnosis of psychosis in people of African origin has been observed with Jamaican immigrants in the United Kingdom.

Associating immigration with poor mental health. Another possible example of pernicious ethnocentric perspectives is the negative view held in the United States during the nineteenth and twentieth centuries on the mental health status of early immigrants to North America, which led to the belief that immigrants had higher levels of mental disorders.[13]

The mental health consequences of migration have been debated in American psychiatry since the end of the nineteenth century, a time when the immigrant pool started to shift from English and Central European set-tlers to those from Southern and Eastern Europe. New immigrants were often characterized as "mental defectives." Many of the reports during the first half of the twentieth century continued to emphasize the mental health disadvantages of the foreign-born compared to the well-assimilated groups.[14] Indeed, immigrants were more frequently institutionalized in state hospital systems compared to the U.S.-born, and were diagnosed as suffering from psychotic disorders much more frequently.[15] At the time, there was a belief that the process of acculturation (melting pot) would dispel many of these problems.

The Abuse of Psychiatry during the Francoist Regime in Spain

To provide an important historical example whose impact is still being felt, we present here a well-documented but little-known account of psychiatric abuse that we believe is rather unique. It involved the use of mainstream academic psychiatry in Spain that was embedded in Francisco Franco's totalitarian establishment for the purpose of labeling, isolating, and ultimately imprisoning and murdering thousands of people from the opposition (Republicans, socialists, communists). What makes this particular instance different and more salient than other global abuses of psychiatry is that interventions were justified on the basis of a well-articulated theory and body of "research," and that the key psychiatrist leading the implementation of these actions, Antonio Vallejo-Nágera, a leading Spanish psychiatrist, would eventually reach the highest academic post and have significant influence on psychiatric theory and education in Spain.

Background. A family friend of Francisco Franco and his wife, Carmen-Polo, Vallejo-Nágera was named director of military and psychiatric services under Franco during the outbreak of the Spanish Civil War in the summer of 1936. The war was fought between the Republicans, those loyal to Spain's democratic and nonsectarian Spanish Republic, and the Nationalists, the fascist rebel group led by Franco. The democratic government of Spain was established on April 14, 1931, after the fall of the dictatorship of Miguel Primo de Rivera and the abdication of King Alfonso XIII. The Spanish Civil War began with a July 1936 rebellion led by a group of politically conservative army officers called *Africanistas,* a term applied to those Spaniards that held posts in the Spanish Army of Africa, which guarded Spain's colonial possessions on that continent. The officers were displeased with the progressive reforms of the new republic, especially the separation of church and state, and were ultimately driven to rebellion. Franco and Vallejo-Nágera were both Africanistas. Franco would ultimately lead the Nationalist movement and name Vallejo-Nágera as director of military and psychiatric services.[16] What is most curious regarding Vallejo-Nágera's new position is the question of the post itself, "director of military and psychiatric services." What was the significance of this position? In what way would a psychiatrist play a significant role in Franco's dictatorship? As demonstrated in the global examples listed above, the variety of diagnoses, the variability of clinical presentations, and the use of specific diagnostic criteria made the use of psychiatry an attractive science in the stigmatization and denigration of Franco's opposition.

To Vallejo-Nágera, political opposition to Franco's military insurgency was conflated with a sense of biological inferiority. Much like the label of "sluggish schizophrenia" and others employed by the USSR, the Nationalist movement had also crafted a new language of political discourse based upon a "remaking of the *patria* (homeland) through the destruction of all things foreign or alien to the 'national destiny.'"[16] Specific language targeting *ofensores de la patria* (offenders of the homeland) was adopted to characterize those loyal to Spain's democratic republic, an inferior race and a danger to the core values of the state. An accomplished medical doctor and military psychiatrist, Vallejo-Nágera published extensively throughout Spain on this topic, writing about the Spanish Civil War through the lens of psychiatric health, and the threat posed by the mentally degenerate Republican enemy.

In their role as professionals highly regarded by the public, medical doctors became politicized figures in the course of the war. As Michael Richards writes, "Although there was no simple ideological divide amongst doctors, the fact that medical doctors ranked high amongst the professional groups targeted in the political violence on both sides underlined the politicization of medicine and medical discourse."[17] Even before accepting his new post in Franco's regime, Vallejo-Nágera had written of his political conservatism as a physician, conflating it with better medical practice. In his book *Divagaciones intrascendentes*, a collection of nine essays published between October 1935 and April 1936, he writes of the ideal physician as Catholic, conservative, and in opposition to Spain's Second Republic (1931–1939). He writes, "El medico debe tener ideas políticas . . . Incluso a la cabecera de la cama del enfermo debe el medico hacer política, claro está que si se entiende por política mantener una ideología que beneficie al individuo y a la comunidad."[18] Here, Vallejo argues that Spanish physicians should bear their political ideas at the bedside of the sick, maintaining an ideology that benefits the individual and the community. Vallejo-Nágera agreed with Franco that the Second Spanish Republic, with its progressive reforms, presented a danger to the Spanish state, positing that it produced less competent physicians. In appointing Vallejo-Nágera, Franco saw a manner by which to delegitimize liberal medical practices that stood at odds with his regime.

Like Cuban eugenicists Angel Arce and José Chelala Aguilera, Vallejo-Nágera believed in the importance of the sexual education of the race. In his

1938 book *Política racial del nuevo estado* (*Racial Politic of the New State*), he
writes of his vision for the regeneration of the Spanish race as a hierarchical
and eugenic state that values Catholicism and gives allegiance to Franco as
dictator. The content of each of the book's sixteen chapters varies consider-
ably, ranging from the importance of marriage and the danger of being an
unmarried woman, to the importance of sexual education and a campaign
against the illnesses of hysteria and neurasthenia.[19]

Similar to Angel Arce in Cuba, who believed that the responsibility of
sexual education fell upon the government, Antonio Vallejo-Nágera had a
similar vision. Sexual education in Spain centered upon an antipornography
campaign, the exercise of sexual self-restraint or continence until marriage,
monogamy, and the absence of sexual perversion. The responsibility for education fell not only upon parents and teachers but upon the Catholic Church
as well, a reflection of the intimate ties between Francoism and Catholicism.
Again, in his text *Política racial del nuevo estado*, Vallejo-Nágera employs a well-
crafted metaphor to relay the dangers of straying from the archetype of the
idealized, pious, Spanish citizen, this time in the form of a spoiled egg:

> No queremos ocurra en España con la higiene racial lo que nos sucedió en cierta
> ocasión con un huevo pasado por agua, que pedimos en un renombrado res-
> taurante de lujo. Un huevo de extraordinario tamaño, de limpia y nacarada
> cáscara, presentada en argentada huevera, pero que encontramos putrefacto.
> La política racial del nuevo estado ha de ser fresca, nutritiva y jugosa para la
> raza, nunca empollada ni podrida.[20]

> In the case of racial hygiene, we do not want to see happening in Spain what
> happened to us in one occasion, when in a renowned restaurant we ordered a
> soft-boiled egg. An egg of extraordinary size, with a clean and pearly shell, was
> presented in a silver egg cup, but we found it to be putrefied. The racial politic
> of the new state must be fresh, nutritious, and juicy for the race, never hatched
> or rotten.

To Vallejo-Nágera, the seemingly large and pearly egg in the silver cup is
Spain, a nation with the traditional values of Catholicism, patriotism, and
self-sufficiency, and the inner putrefaction is the damage done to the traditional values by the Spanish Republic, with its progressive reforms separating
church and state, legalizing divorce, and allowing for secular education.

Vallejo-Nágera's *racial politic*, his idealized state not tainted by progressive reform and secularism, will save the egg from spoiling, allowing it to remain fresh, nutritious, and juicy.[18]

As historian Ricard Vinyes reflects on Vallejo-Nágera's use of the term "race,"

> En la cabeza de Vallejo la expresion *raza* poseía un carácter singular. Nada que ver con las tesis biológicas de franceses, británicos o alemanes. Singular porque la raza no correspondía a un grupo biológico humano sino a una sociedad-la de la época de la caballería-, a un grupo social-la aristocracia- y una forma de gobierno fundamentada en la disciplina militar y depositaria de unas presumibles virtudes patrióticas destruidas por el sentido plebeyo de la burguesía y las clases bajas.[21]

> In Vallejo's head, the expression "race" had a singular character. It had nothing to do with the biological theses of the French, British, or Germans. Its character was singular because his concept of race did not correspond to a human biological group but to a society—that of the age of chivalry—to a social group—the aristocracy—and a form of government based on military discipline which was the depository of presumable patriotic virtues destroyed by the plebeian sense of the bourgeoisie and the lower classes.

By Vallejo-Nágera's characterization, the true dangers brought by the Spanish Second Republic were not related to a sectarian perspective or to promoting the rights of women; rather, the Republicans by nature were anti-Spanish. In this sense, he regarded the enemy not solely as a political or social adversary but as a destructive and inhumane force from which the country needed to be freed. In his 1938 publication *Divagaciones intrascendentes*, Vallejo-Nágera writes, "Mi patria ha sufrido grandes catástrofes, inmensas desgracias, perdió su poderío, se ha empobrecido; pero amo a mi patria desgraciada y pobre y trabajaré para que vuelva a ser feliz, rica, poderosa, respetada y temida."[18] (My country has suffered great catastrophes, immense misfortunes, lost its power, has become impoverished; but I love my poor and disgraced country, and I will work to make her happy, rich, powerful, respected, and feared.) Vallejo-Nágera's statement is clearly a political one; however, its emphasis is not on the enemy itself but on the nation whose *traditional values* have been destroyed. The focus upon the powerful and respected nation in contrast to the poor and disgraced nonnation together form a discourse of elimination, characteristic of extreme right political ideology, and seen across much of Vallejo-Nágera's work. Also notable is Vallejo-Nágera's personification of the Spanish state, as he ascribes to it qualities it must reacquire, including happiness, power, and respect.[18]

Perhaps most telling in this text is Vallejo-Nágera's use of metaphor to communicate to readers the danger of the Republican enemy ascending the social hierarchy. To Vallejo-Nágera and to Franco, only Nationalists should occupy professional posts, and the Republicans should be repressed; any challenge to the regime would not be tolerated. With this point in mind, Vallejo-Nágera writes that the selection of career must correspond with the individual's place in the social and eugenic hierarchy of Spain, and that children should adopt the careers of their parents. In explaining these principles, Vallejo-Nágera introduces his metaphor, relating the story of a young medical doctor who upon completing years of training returns to his small village to pursue his true passion: working in the confectionary owned by his father.[19] Vallejo-Nágera writes,

> No es el único caso que podríamos referir de personas que después de sacrificar años y caudales en costosa carrera, han de tornar a la profesión de los padres, en la que prosperan y nunca debieron abandonar. Es peligroso para el Estado y para la Sociedad que el hijo del comerciante o del industrial ejerza profesiones liberales, porque suele mercantilizarlas.[20]

This is not the only case that could refer to those people who, after sacrificing years and costs in an expensive career, have returned to the profession of their parents, in which they thrive and should never have left. It is dangerous for the state and for society that the son of a merchant or an industrialist exercises a liberal profession, as it tends to commodify him.

Vallejo-Nágera's anecdote regarding this medical doctor who should never have left his father's candy shop is significant in the sense that the Nationalists viewed the education and upward social mobility of the enemy as dangerous to their own cause. This young man, who presumably is from a poor town and is the son of an uneducated merchant, is not the man who Franco's regime envisions attending medical school. In keeping with the eugenic hierarchy, the man should remain in his father's shop throughout his working life; in this way, he will not become well educated nor begin to question the regime that silences his people.

Case report. As a writer skilled in the use of metaphor, Vallejo-Nágera published prolifically throughout the Spanish Civil War, in publications targeted both for the medical community and for the general public. Up to 1938, at the time of the release of *Política racial del nuevo estado*, however, Vallejo-Nágera had written largely of the threat of the Republican enemy to the Nationalist movement. Vallejo-Nágera had not, to this point, experimented on imprisoned Republican subjects. The year 1938 was a pivotal one for the Franco regime, with the creation of a formal Cabinet of Psychological Investigation authorized by Franco on August 23, 1938, with the stated purpose of investigating "las raíces psicofísicas del marxismo" (the psychophysical roots of Marxism).[22] In its first year, the cabinet published the results of its first study on political prisoners simultaneously in two Spanish medical journals: *Semana Médica Española* and *Revista Española de Cirugía y Medicina de Guerra*.

This notable study, "Psyche of Marxist Fanaticism: Psychologic Investigations on Delinquent Marxist Feminists," was conducted on fifty female political prisoners jailed in a provincial prison in Málaga, Spain. From a scientific perspective, this was far from being a sound research study, as the methodology included a 200-item questionnaire administered to the women, we assume, under duress. Other than administering psychological tests assessing IQ (Binet Simon) and temperament (Neyman-Kohlsted, a test used to assess introversion or extroversion), there were no systematic physical or psychiatric assessments to support the purported "psychiatric degeneracy" of the Republican women.

The results from the study are detailed in a number of tables, including demographics, personal information, individual beliefs, prison sentence and associated crimes, primary temperament, intelligence, level of education, economic position, profession, religious and political beliefs, and opinions on the political regime. In his 1986 autobiographical book *Prisoners of the Good Fight*, Carl Geiser, an American International Brigadier imprisoned by the Franco regime reflected upon his own imprisonment and a similar questionnaire that he was forced to complete as an imprisoned man: "They had a two hundred-item questionnaire in English, German, French and Spanish. It began with name, race and nationality, education, skills, jobs held, criminal record, family income, names and addresses of relatives, then came political and social questions, then ethical questions, including religious affiliation and beliefs and finally, our views on free love, and the questions: 'When did you first have sexual intercourse? With whom?'"[23] Following the presentation of each set of survey questions and the individual responses to them, there are a number of blanket statements both praising the regime and dehumanizing the women as perverse and threatening to the core values of the Spanish state. This study is significant, as it provides insight into Francoist eugenic theory and the means by which members of the medical community defended the imprisonment and murder of thousands of Spanish citizens.

As a starting point in the discussion, Vallejo-Nágera defends the exclusion of the physical examination of the patient because "en el sexo femenino, esto carece de finalidad, por la impureza de los contornos" (in the female gender, this lacks purpose due to the impurity of their contours).[24]

With the goal of establishing a dichotomy between the kind, subservient, and religious Francoist woman, and the "degenerate, infantilized and even animalistic Republican woman," Vallejo-Nágera concludes that the moral degeneracy of Republicanism constitutes a threat to the Spanish state. To Vallejo-Nágera, the imprisoned Republican women stand in stark contrast to those women who comprised the female branch of the Spanish fascist party, the Sección Femenina (Feminine Section). Pilar Primo de Rivera, sister of Spanish Falange Party founder José Antonio Primo de Rivera, founded the Sección Femenina in 1936.[25] Far from a party in name only, the group played an important role in the Franco regime throughout the Spanish Civil War. Its senior members (*mandos*) ensured that women throughout the Spanish state were fulfilling the proper and traditional role of women in society, namely, raising a traditionalist family loyal to the regime. Sexism was inherent within the regime, and despite the significant role that these women served in furthering the ideals of the dictatorship, their role was always lesser in importance to that of men. In her 1938 speech to the Second National Congress of the Sección Femenina of the Falange Española Tradicionalista (FET) y de las Juntas de Ofensiva Nacional Sindicalista (JONS), Pilar Primo de Rivera remarked, "Lo que no haremos nunca es ponerlas en competencia con ellos, porque jamás llegarán a igualarnos, y en cambio, pierden toda la elegancia y toda la gracia indispensable para la convivencia."[26] (What we will never do is have the women compete with the men, as they will never equal us, and instead, in doing so, they lose the elegance and the grace so indispensable to their existence.)

The objectification of Republican females and the violence enacted upon them was based upon the principle of "gynephobia," a fear and rejection of those not adhering to the archetypal fascist female.[19] As Hispanist scholar Timothy Mitchell discusses, the practice of medicine during the Franco regime was so heavily controlled by the Catholic Church and the Falange that only the most politically and religiously devout, such as Vallejo-Nágera, rose to positions of power. In his description of the idealized Fascist woman, Mitchell writes, "It was recommended that she be of medium height, with hips slightly wider than her shoulders, smooth skin, and well-developed breasts. Women were understood to be weak, more or less passive, more or less perverse, particularly vulnerable to psychosomatic illness, clearly unstable. Spanish gynecological treatises of the epoch were resolutely opposed to women working outside the home: not only did it contribute to the 'corruption of customs' and the 'destruction of family,' it was a major cause of disease."[27]

With the image of the idealized Republican woman in mind, the goal of the regime was to violently repress any woman not fitting with the description above, and to indoctrinate the rest in the ways of political and social obedience. Beginning in 1941, the women of the Sección Femenina served the regime by taking part in the *cuerpo de divulgación*, a voluntary community-level volunteer healthcare project in which women would educate their neighbors on such topics as the illegality of abortion, the need to choose a healthy partner if considering marriage, and the merits of state-sponsored healthcare.[25] In many ways, the female *cuerpo de divulgación* teams served to enforce the eugenic principles espoused by Vallejo-Nágera's teachings, among them an allegiance to Franco and a rejection of all that was Republican and thus anti-Spanish.[25]

Language played a particularly important role for the regime in describing the supposed degeneracy of the Republican woman, perhaps best evidenced by one of the subtitles within the publication *Material Studied*, which details the demographics of the women included in the research. After relaying the prison sentence of each woman—66 percent received the death sentence—Vallejo-Nágera writes that "la magnanimidad del Caudillo ha conmutado las penas de muerte por la de reclusion perpetua en todos los casos que estudiamos"[24] (the magnanimity of our leader has commuted the death sentences to that of life sentences in all cases studied). Here, Vallejo-Nágera characterizes Franco as a magnanimous and benevolent leader, whose kindness has lessened the sentences of thirty-three of the fifty women to terms of life imprisonment. In reality, the act is hardly magnanimous, as the women are guilty of no crime apart from their political affiliation. The article makes no mention of specific crimes being equated with corresponding sentences, citing offenses only in vague terms such as "rebellion and other political crimes."[24]

Vallejo-Nágera's section concerning the religious beliefs of the imprisoned women, and his accompanying commentary, are also quite telling. After mentioning that five of the fifty women are pious, sixteen are practicing, fifteen are nonpracticing, thirteen are indifferent, and one is atheist, Vallejo-Nágera concludes that despite the majority of women being Catholic, their "religious ideas are limited to a vague and confusing sentiment that admits the existence of God."[24] When faced with survey findings consistent with his own beliefs of the idealized Spanish state (i.e., high rates of Catholic citizens), Vallejo-Nágera resorts to a poorly substantiated and confusing claim questioning the true sentiment of these women. This example further highlights the inadequacy of the survey in demonstrating the supposed psychiatric inferiority of these women.

In the final section of the study, Vallejo-Nágera examines the political beliefs of the imprisoned women. One question asked of the woman is "What is your opinion of Nationalist Spain?" with 48 percent having a good opinion, 14 percent claiming it was a better organized system than the democratic regime, 2 percent stating that they must wait to form an opinion, 30 percent responding that they were unsure, and 4 percent expressing a poor opinion. In the accompanying commentary, Vallejo-Nágera asserts that the good opinion the prisoners have of the regime stems from the fact that despite being enemies, the regime cares for their children, protects the poor, and provides work, in contrast to the claims of the opposition's "red propaganda." Next, he defends the 30 percent response from those who were unsure of their opinion because they have been imprisoned and have not experienced the magnanimity of the regime firsthand. Lastly, the few women with a poor opinion of the regime appear to be referring actually to their personal situation and not the nation as a whole.

In claiming that the regime cares for the children of its Republican enemies, Vallejo-Nágera is likely referring to the Prisión de Madres Lactantes, or Prison of Lactating Mothers, in Madrid. In this and similar facilities, mothers and nursing children were physically separated for twenty-three hours a day, with most women ultimately being killed or remaining in prison after being stripped of their children. These children were given to devoutly Catholic parents loyal to the regime.[28] In this sense, Vallejo-Nágera's claims of caring for the children of the enemy may largely be discredited.

CONCLUSIONS

The example of Antonio Vallejo-Nágera and the abuse of psychiatry in Francoist Spain is unique in its intimate tie between psychiatry and politics and the establishment of a chief of psychiatric services for the regime.[29] The detention, imprisonment, and even murder of members of the Republican opposition were defended by medical doctors in medical journals and bulletins as a necessary step in the cleansing of the Spanish state, in keeping with the core Nationalist values of religion, patriotism, and self-sufficiency.

The abuse of psychiatry has a long and far-reaching global history, with the rich lexicon of psychiatric diagnoses and variable diagnostic criteria functioning as a dangerous language of stigmatization and repression at the hands of the ruling class, government, or regime. As has been demonstrated in this chapter, falsified or wrongly attributed psychiatric diagnoses have been applied to innocent individuals throughout history with the goal of objectification, imprisonment, or even murder. While many psychiatric abuses, such as those in Francoist Spain, are from an earlier historical time, the example of the abuse of the Falun Gong religious sect in China took place only in the last twenty years. Because psychiatric abuse is far from an issue of the past, it is important that physicians continue to act in the best interests of their patients and honor the principle of non-maleficence.

REFERENCE LIST

1. Burleigh M. Surveys of developments in the social history of medicine: III: "Euthanasia" in the Third Reich: Some recent literature. *Social History of Medicine*. 1991;4(2): 317–328. https://doi.org/10.1093/shm/4.2.317.
2. Luty J. Psychiatry and the dark side: Eugenics, Nazi and Soviet psychiatry." *Advances in Psychiatric Treatment*. 2014;20(1):52–60. https://doi.org/10.1192/apt.bp.112.010330.
3. Van Voren R. Political abuse of psychiatry—An historical overview." *Schizophrenia Bulletin*. 2009;36(1):33–35. https://doi.org/10.1093/schbul/sbp119.

4. Kent A. Dangerous minds: Political psychiatry in China today and its origins in the Mao era. *China Quarterly*. 2003;176. https://doi.org/10.1017/s0305741003250633.

5. Munro R. Judicial psychiatry in China and its political abuses. *Columbia Journal of Asian Law*. 2000;14(1):1–128.

6. Arvey S. Sex and the ordinary Cuban: Cuban physicians, eugenics, and marital sexuality, 1933–1958. *Journal of the History of Sexuality*. 2012;21(1):93–120. https://doi.org/10 .1353/sex.2012.0004.

7. Arce A. *El problema sexual y social de Cuba: El hombre ignorante sexual* Alerta, La Habana, 1956.

8. Fernando S. Race and culture issues in mental health and some thoughts on ethnic identity. *Counseling Psychology Quarterly*. 2012;25(2):113–123.

9. Fernando S. *Race and Culture in Psychiatry*. New York: Routledge; 2016.

10. Szasz TS. The sane slave. *American Journal of Psychotherapy*. 1971;25(2):228–239. https://doi.org/10.1176/appi.psychotherapy.1971.25.2.228.

11. Strakowski SM, Shelton RC, Kolbrener ML. The effects of race and comorbidity on clinical diagnoses in patients with psychosis. *Journal of Clinical Psychiatry*. 1993;54:96–102.

12. Minsky S, William V, Miskimen T, Gara M, Escobar J. Diagnostic patterns in Latino, African American, and European American psychiatric patients. *Archives of General Psychiatry*. 2003;60(6):637–644. https://doi.org/10.1001/archpsyc.60.6.637.

13. Oodegard O. A statistical investigation of the incidence of mental disorder in Norway. *Psychiatric Quarterly*. 1945;20(3):382–383. https://doi.org/10.1007/bf01574330.

14. Malzberg B. Mental disease among native- and foreign-born whites in New York State. *Mental Hygiene*. 1964;48:478–499.

15. Srole L, Langner TS, Michael SI, Opler M, Rennie TAC. Mental health in the metropolis: The midtown Manhattan study. *American Journal of Sociology*. 1968;73(4):528–529.

16. Richards M. *A Time of Silence: Civil War and the Culture of Repression in Franco's Spain, 1936–1945*. Cambridge: Cambridge University Press; 1998.

17. Richards M. Spanish psychiatry c. 1900–1945: Constitutional theory, eugenics, and the nation. *Bulletin of Spanish Studies*. 2004;81(6):823–848.

18. Vallejo-Nágera A. *Divagaciones Intrascendentes*. Valladolid: Talleres Tipográficos Cuesta; 1938.

19. Pearlstein EF. Antonio Vallejo-Nágera and the discourse of eugenics in Francoist Spain. W&M ScholarWorks. 2015. https://publish.wm.edu/honorstheses/146/.

20. Vallejo-Nágera A. *Política racial del nuevo estado*. San Sebastian: Editorial Española; 1938.

21. Ribas RV. Construyendo a Caín Diagnosis y terapia del disidente: Las investigaciones psiquiátricas militares de Antonio Vallejo-Nágera con presas y presos políticos. *Ayer*. 2001;44:227–250.

22. Carvallo de Cora E. *Hoja de servicios del Caudillo de España Don Francisco Franco Bahamonde, y su genealogia*. Madrid; 1967.

23. Geiser C. *Prisoners of the Good Fight: The Spanish Civil War, 1936–1939*. Westport, Conn.: Lawrence Hill; 1986.

24. Vallejo-Nágera A, Martínez E. Psiquismo del fanatismo marxista. Investigaciones psicológicas en marxistas femeninos delincuentes. *Revista Española de medicina y cirugía de guerra.* 1939;9:398–413.

25. Richmond K. *Women and Spanish Fascism: The Women's Section of the Falange, 1934–1959.* London: Routledge; 2003.

26. Domingo C. Discurso de Pilar Primo de Rivera en El II Congreso Nacional de la Sección Femenina de FET y de las JONS (Segovia, 1938). In: *Nosotras también hicimos la guerra: Defensoras y sublevadas.* Barcelona: Flor del Viento Ediciones; 2006.

27. Mitchell TJ. Authoritarian medicalization and gynephobia under Franco. *South Central Review.* 2004;21(2):1–14.

28. Pérez J, Vinyes R, Armengou M, Belis R. Los niños perdidos del franquismo. *Hispania.* 2005;88(4):764. https://doi.org/10.2307/20063190.

29. Pearlstein E, Escobar JI. Antonio Vallejo-Nágera (1889–1960) and Juan Antonio Vallejo-Nágera Botas (1926–1990). *American Journal of Psychiatry.* 2018;175(8):720–722. https://doi.org/10.1176/appi.ajp.2018.18020155.

4 · TASK-SHIFTING STRATEGIES IN LATIN AMERICA

The Key Role of Primary Care Health Agents in Mental Health Policy and Research in Northern Argentina

MARIA CALVO, GABRIEL DE ERAUSQUIN, MARIANA FIGUEREDO AGUIAR, EDUARDO PADILLA, AND JAVIER I. ESCOBAR

In this chapter, we describe an ongoing global mental health collaboration targeting psychotic disorders. A major focus of the chapter is to highlight a "task-shifting" strategy successfully used to support a research program targeting the identification of subjects with severe mental disorders, particularly schizophrenia, in the region of Jujuy in northern Argentina. This strategy involved multiple layers of collaboration—locally, nationally, and internationally—aimed at developing local research capacity, establishing technology-based collaboration tools, and acquiring, storing, sharing, and publishing high-quality data with the appropriate ethical and privacy safeguards. Implementation of this research initiative required the creation of an international consortium that included investigators from leading institutions in the United States, the United Kingdom, and the South American countries of Peru, Argentina, and Bolivia. This consortium mentored and trained a local team that included mental health professionals (psychiatrists, psychologists). However, the central element and key innovation of this consortium was the training of primary care health agents for the tasks of identifying, referring for assessment, and helping with the management of individuals with severe mental health problems. All these tasks were performed under the supervision of and in continuous coordination with research psychiatrists and psychologists based at the provincial capital's neuropsychiatric hospital.

This capacity-building process resulted in measurable improvements in several health outcomes for individuals with severe mental disorders. It facilitated and improved access to the primary health care system, influenced needed changes in local health policy, and made important scientific contributions to mainstream psychiatry. One of these contributions was the recognition of the neurological component (movement disorders) that often accompanies the psychotic syndromes of neuroleptic-naïve patients with schizophrenia.

THE RESEARCH SETTING

The research was performed in Jujuy, Northern Argentina. The province of Jujuy, Argentina is located in the Andean Mountains next to the borders of Bolivia and Chile. It has 672,307 inhabitants, unevenly distributed across urban and rural areas.

Most of Jujuy's population is aboriginal, with the highest concentration of first nation communities located in the mountains, where most people belong to the Kechwa (*colla*) ethnocultural group. The province presents unique geographical characteristics (Figure 4.1), combining rainforest (*yunga*), flat, productive highlands (*valles*), and isolated, high mountainous areas (*quebrada* and *puna*). The highest population density is found in the valleys, where the capital city, San Salvador de Jujuy, with an estimated 350,000 inhabitants, is located. There are also several smaller towns with economies based on agriculture and mining. The area of the Yungas ("rainforest" in the local dialect), occupies the eastern slopes of the Andes Mountains. It has a warm and humid climate and a few population centers and small towns that are fairly isolated. In fact, many of these communities may often get completely

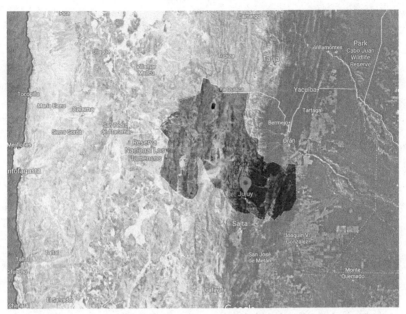

FIGURE 4.1. Satellite image of the Province of Jujuy, Argentina. The Eastern end of the territory (dark gray) is the rainforest region or "yungas." The Western side of the Province (light gray) consists of dry highlands and mountain ranges, or "quebrada" and "puna." The location marker signals the capital city of San Salvador, and the area to its South marks the productive highlands region or "valles."

isolated during the rainy seasons. These communities are located far away from hospitals and health care centers. The Eastern mountainous region includes the "Quebrada" and "Puna" . It is a mountainous area that has the lowest population density in the region, with small villages some of which are only accessible by foot or by horseback and have as few as twenty inhabitants living in isolated family dwellings. The Puna suffers from extreme seasonal variations of temperature and humidity and has scarce vegetation. Rural inhabitants in these regions of the province often have significant difficulties accessing resources due to the mountainous terrain, jungles, and poor road infrastructure. The northwestern region of the province, which has the lowest population density in the province, is the primary focus of this report.

The history of the primary health care agents (PHCAs) in the province of Jujuy starts with Carlos Alberto Alvarado, the pioneer for implementing health and mental health programs in the region. Born in San Salvador de Jujuy in 1908, Alvarado led the successful efforts for eradication of malaria

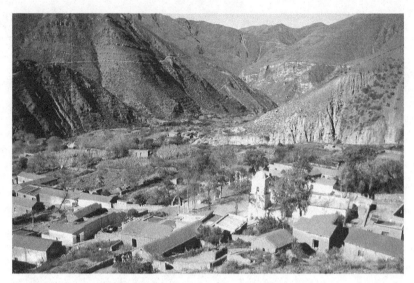

FIGURE 4.2. Town of Caspala, in the "Quebrada" region. The town has a population of less than 200, no cellular phone tower within reach, and only one CB radio station used by the local Primary Care Health Agent to contact the Province emergency services in case of need. The only road connecting the town with the rest of the province is made of consolidated dirt and ends about 1 mile away from the town. Two individuals with chronic, unmedicated psychosis were identified here after the onset of IMAGES. The town health agent became responsible for their follow up, management of medication adhesion, and report/referral of relapses back to the treating team in the capital.

in Argentina in 1945 while working for the National Ministry of Health, and globally as chief of the coordination office of the Malaria Eradication Program of the World Health Organization.[1] As early as 1938, Alvarado had already emphasized the need for prevention of mental illness (psychosis) and the importance of research.[2] Upon returning to his native Argentina, he served as health minister of the province of Jujuy and designed the Rural Health Plan in 1966, a visionary strategy that anticipated the declaration at Alma Ata in 1978[3] and formalized the strategy of primary health care as a policy, bringing health closer to the people, with the slogan "House by house, person by person." Alvarado stated that Argentina "counts on eminent doctors specialized in diseases" and that "the country needs medical specialists in health, to conserve and improve health."[3] He proposed a plan for the region that included the following elements:

- Protection of maternity and childhood (outside of hospitals)
- Hygiene of the child and adolescent (physical, mental, and moral)
- Diets that satisfy all the physiological needs of the human body, for its growth and conservation of health
- Cleaning, lighting, ventilating, and heating of households and work environments
- Prevention of noncommunicable diseases (cancer, heart disease, psychosis, etc.)
- Health education and hygiene propaganda
- Epidemiology (statistics on health and healthcare)
- Research in health and healthcare

A key element of the Rural Health Plan was the introduction of community health workers, now called primary care health agents (PCHAs). PCHAs are persons who belong to a community, receive training in various health areas such as vaccines or the importance of pregnancy control, and have the specific responsibility to visit a number of assigned households each year with the main purpose of surveying and assessing their compliance with vaccination plans and other health initiatives. However, at the time of the project's initiation, the role of the PCHAs did not include a mental health component. Therefore, the initial strategy was the systematic training of these PCHAs for the initial recognition of people who might be suffering from mental symptoms, and the design of an efficient system of communication with mental health specialists similar to the "task-shifting" system proposed by the WHO.[4]

Primary care services in the Region of Jujuy are provided by the Ministry of Health System (MHS). The MHS secures virtual universal access to basic care without any direct cost to consumers. The MHS is divided into six administrative/geographical areas and is built on a system centered around three tertiary care hospitals in San Salvador de Jujuy, including one general acute hospital, one children's hospital, and one neuropsychiatric hospital. There are also six medium-size rural hospitals (one in each region); twenty-six small community hospitals providing such services as prenatal care, labor and delivery, and basic surgery; and 242 primary health care centers (CAPS in the Spanish acronym) providing ambulatory and preventive services. Traditionally, MHS general practitioners and primary care nurses did not receive formal training in mental health, and this became an additional barrier to mental health care in the region. While licensed psychologists with training in community mental health are available at community hospitals and provide mental health assessments and psychotherapy, they are not qualified or authorized to manage pharmacotherapy. The few psychiatrists working for the MHS are based at the neuropsychiatric hospital in San Salvador de Jujuy. Therefore, consultations by mental health specialists are only available at this facility.

The MHS thus relies heavily on the PCHAs who are responsible for health surveillance through periodic home visits. The PCHAs are recruited in their communities as full-time employees of the MHS. They have a high school education and receive specific training focused on surveillance and prevention of communicable diseases and other primary care health tasks such as prenatal care and vaccination campaigns. The PCHAs serve as the link between community dwellers and their medical providers, and through their home visits, they become the central point of entry into the MHS. Approximately 800 PCHAs cover the entire territory of the region and visit each household at least once per year. During these periodic visits, PCHAs provide health education, collect health data, assess compliance with prevention campaigns, provide medications prescribed by physicians, and help with laboratory testing. Moreover, they facilitate access to higher levels of health care through referrals and transportation arrangements.

THE RESEARCH OPPORTUNITY

Until 2002, the training of community health workers in the province of Jujuy had focused on surveillance, referral and management of transmissible diseases (such as tuberculosis, Chagas disease, and dengue fever), and other primary care health concerns (such as prenatal care and vaccination campaigns). Since no specific training on mental health was provided to these workers, numerous individuals with psychiatric conditions were never identified or referred for appropriate evaluation and treatment, except in cases of violence or acute agitation. This resulted in protracted durations of severe untreated mental illness. Thus, there was a unique opportunity for a new research initiative aimed at studying severe mental disorders among subjects whose illness had not yet been properly recognized and who were therefore unexposed to psychiatric medications. The intervention strategy was to train existing community health workers on the identification, referral, and follow-up for individuals suffering from these severe disorders. An ambitious plan was therefore outlined to implement an innovative system for detection of untreated mental disorders in rural areas of the province and to assess its impact on the duration of untreated psychosis. Another goal was to evaluate the psychiatric and neurologic phenomenology of chronic psychotic disorders on individuals with chronic psychotic disorders who were not exposed to psychotropic medications early in the course of their illness, and to examine the heritability of movement disorders in this unique population.

THE STUDY IMAGES

The study Investigation of Movement Abnormalities and the Genetics of Schizophrenia (IMAGES) was originally piloted using funds provided by the Brain and Behavior Research Foundation. The research continued to be supported with funds from this foundation as well as other funding agencies, including the National Institutes of Health (NIH) during the period 2002 to 2016.

In approaching the task of developing a health research and intervention program, a serious problem in countries like Argentina is the lack of epidemiological data, especially in the most impoverished provinces. At the outset of the IMAGES study, the only available data were scattered statistics on the number of contacts, type of diagnoses, and discharge records of service contacts provided at the hospitals, without any information on community or outpatient attention. On the basis of the number of claims for disability due to schizophrenia in other parts of the region and the country, we inferred that there must be a sizeable number of affected individuals in the more remote areas of the province who had not yet had contact with the health care system. The challenge was then to identify individuals in those remote regions who might be actively suffering from schizophrenia or other major psychoses but who had never been recognized or treated.

IMAGES was based on the premise that a set of neurological motor impairments (e.g., movement disorders) was a marker for the genetic risk of nonaffective psychoses, and that it might be present among at-risk individuals who had never received neuroleptic treatment. The motor impairment was theorized to be present in study subjects and, to some extent, in their first-degree relatives, regardless of the presence of active psychotic symptoms. It was then proposed that the severity of motor impairments would be predictive of the risk and severity of psychiatric disease.

We created and adapted a specific curriculum for training the community health workers on the identification of abnormal behaviors suggestive of severe mental illness, and we developed and implemented a referral process for newly identified cases.[5]

We also implemented a follow-up process, relying on the community health workers to maintain newly identified patients engaged in their care.[5]

To ascertain the psychiatry diagnosis on the new referrals, we used a highly sophisticated clinical instrument, the Schedules for Clinical Assessment in Neuropsychiatry-Present State Examination (SCAN-PSE), a semistructured psychiatric interview developed by the World Health Organization (WHO).[6,7] The WHO had used a previous version of the PSE in the pioneer International Pilot Study of Schizophrenia (IPSS) coordinated in the 1970s.[8] The use of SCAN required specific training and certification of local mental health clinicians (psychologists, psychiatrists) by international experts with experience using the instrument. Assessments of motor functions were videotaped to allow for later scoring by blinded experts and included administration of the Unified Parkinson's Disease Rating Scale (UPDRS)[9] and the Huntington Disease Rating Scale.[10]

In addition, we collected temperament and character descriptions of individual subjects by using the Temperament and Character Inventory (TCI).[11] and obtained profiles of their cognitive performance using a culturally adapted battery specifically designed to minimize the impact of schooling and spoken language on the results.[12]

TRANSLATION AND ADAPTATION OF INSTRUMENTS

The population's native language is Kechwa. Individual and communal perceptions of major mental disorders and their clinical manifestations in Kechwa-speaking populations include a number of unique culturally related terms and idioms.[13] It has been reported that Kechwa healers have a clear conception of the morbid nature of behavioral changes, as denoted by the use of such words as *onqoy*.[14] and that major psychiatric illness can be found in the traditional medical knowledge and practices of the Kechwa of the central Andes, thus highlighting unique "emic" (from phonemics) issues highlighted by traditional cultural psychiatry. Two major reviews of traditional Kechwa medical terminology used to describe psychopathology have been published.[15,16]

All instruments, including the lengthy psychiatric interview (SCAN), were translated into Kechwa and adapted for use in this population with a low socioeconomic and educational background. Prior to the dissemination of Spanish, the dominant language in the Andean region of South America was Kechwa, which remains, to date, the most widely spoken indigenous language in the world. Since Kechwa was not written, much of the existing record of its usage comes through translation by period historians and chroniclers. Much of the traditional medical knowledge has been lost, but current usage frequently retains semantic content with technical implications. The translation of instruments was supervised by Kechwa scholars from Peru and pretested with Kechwa-speaking subjects.

There were other research procedures incorporated as part of the neurological assessment. One of these was the use of transcranial ultrasound to gauge brain changes related to movement disorders. As part of this, we obtained images of the subjects' midbrain area using transcranial ultrasound that measures iron deposition in the substantia nigra. This appears to be a well-accepted, measurable marker for Parkinson's disease that seems to be related to the degree of motor impairment.[17] Also, blood samples were taken for genetic studies. Subjects signed an informed consent (also translated into Kechwa) prior to participating in the research.

The challenging execution of this project required the recruitment of a group of highly competent professionals committed to ongoing research training and to breaking down barriers to mental health care. An interdisciplinary team of psychiatrists, psychologists, neuroimaging specialists, and biologists familiar with the local culture and habits of the population was assembled. International collaborators from leading U.S. and European institutions provided mentoring and assistance with the various aspects of the research.

Training of Health Agents for the Detection, Referral, and Follow-up of Severe Mental Illness: We developed and implemented annual training sessions that were delivered in each major region of the province (Valleys, Yunga, Puna) to all provincial PCHAs (slightly over 200 in each region). Attending the training courses required a great personal effort on the part of the PCHAs,

TABLE 4.1.   Impact of Training on Health Agents' Proficiency to Recognize
Characteristic Psychopathology

	Alcohol	Stimulants	Mania	Psychosis
Pre	47.7	31.4	30.2	37.2
Post	91.7	72.6	1.8	97.2

A survey consisting of vignettes with typical clinical presentations and questions about symptoms more commonly seen in patients with each diagnoses was presented before (pre) and after (post) training day. Surveys were filled anonymously. Cells represent the percent of vignettes correctly identified by the health agents before and after training for each pathological category.

since some of them had to travel large distances on horseback or on foot before reaching public transport stations with connections to the training sites. Often they had to start the trip a day earlier. Each yearly training session was led by psychiatrists and usually lasted three hours. Sessions included presentations on the clinical characteristics and symptoms of severe mental illness, illustrative videos, updates on the research, recognition of performance on the previous year, and unstructured time to discuss local problems and realities of each community and to answer questions and address concerns.

Impact of Training on Health Agents' Proficiency to Recognize Characteristic Signs of Substance Use, Mania, and Psychosis: A survey including vignettes with typical clinical presentations and queries about symptoms commonly seen in these conditions was presented to the PCHAs before and after the training day. Surveys were filled anonymously. As can be seen in table 4.1, the percent of clinical vignettes correctly identified by the PCHAs increased exponentially after the training for each of the four dimensions assessed.

Referral System to Specialty Care and the Research Team: Another priority, as important as the training sessions, was to rely on a simple and efficient communication system to connect PCHAs who identified a person exhibiting psychiatric symptoms with specialty care and the research team. (Referral to specialty care occurred independently of whether the person qualified for or was interested in research participation.) Once subjects were referred, specialists were then responsible for ensuring that each subject would receive specialized medical attention and the healthcare they needed. Finally, individuals with nonaffective psychoses were invited to participate in the ongoing investigation. Some villages had access to telephone communication or radio, but many distant locations did not have these resources. Indeed, several towns did not even have roads or access for motor vehicles. Therefore, a simple card was designed with the necessary data for all individual contacts.

Procedures for Referral and Assessment: Once the psychiatry team was notified of a case, they were responsible for visiting the person in the village of origin (arranged through the PCHA) or arranging transfer to a healthcare center for assessment there. The action taken was decided by the group according to each particular situation following direct communication with the health agent originating the referral, who was best positioned to plan the best strategy. If a visit was arranged in the village, the PCHA accompanied and introduced the psychiatrist to the patient and his or her family, since the PCHA is usually the person that the family trusts. It is important to highlight that although the main objective of the PCHAs' training was to detect possible subjects affected with psychoses (schizophrenia), their yearly training and ongoing supervision by the psychiatry team also included affective disorders, neurodevelopmental disorders, alcoholism, and suicide risk. Agents were trained to ensure attention to all the mental health needs of the people in their jurisdiction, whether or not they participated in the study.

Another essential element of the success of the initiative was the exclusive focus of the training sessions on mental health issues, enabling the necessary time for PCHAs to concentrate their attention and dedication on this topic. A common alternative strategy is to organize training sessions before the compulsory PCHA meetings. During those sessions, a broad strokes update of all the programs and areas of the Ministry of Health occurs. Competing for delivery of information and requesting attention to interests concerning a great variety of health topics, it results in an excessive amount of data for attendees without allowing adequate time to process and learn or develop new skills. In contrast, our focused training sessions occurred in isolation and were specifically designed to engage attendees' attention on mental health issues and to allow them to acquire and implement new skills.

Health Policy and Institutional Impact: An important element in this regard was the yearly recurrence of training and its inclusion as a continuous educational strategy of the Ministry of Health, with the goal of eventually influencing health policy. Indeed, the provincial health system significantly benefited from the incorporation of mental health strategies into the routines of PCHAs' home visits. These benefits included implementation of a referral and follow-up system for specialty care, and development of a continuous education mental health curriculum for the primary care level. Implementation of this task-shifting system for mental health care contributed to improved accessibility and quality of care for this most vulnerable population. In addition, local research capacity was developed and supported through active and engaged mentorship, resulting in additional research projects with independent funding supported by national and international agencies. A good example of this development of capacity was the proposal "Funding and implementation of the first plan for monitoring and prodromal symptoms of psychosis in populations at risk and a plan for an early detection and treatment of psychoses," which was funded by the National Ministry of Health of Argentina. Of note, the proposal was the first of its kind in the country.

From the institutional point of view, IMAGES acted as the starting point and facilitator for multiple research agreements, mentoring relationships, and student and faculty exchanges between local researchers in the Ministry of Health of Jujuy, and Rutgers University–Robert Wood Johnson Medical School, the Washington University School of Medicine, the University of South Florida, Harvard Medical School, the University of Texas Rio Grande Valley, the University of Leicester (United Kingdom), Universidad Peruana Cayetano Heredia (Peru), Universidad de Buenos Aires and Universidad Technological Nacional de Argentina (Argentina), Universidad Nacional de Asuncion (Paraguay), and Pontificia Universidad San Francisco Javier de Chuquisaca (Bolivia).

In addition, a new not-for-profit organization, Fundación de Lucha contra los Trastornos Neurologicos y Psiquiatricos en Minorias (FULTRA), was created in Argentina for the purpose of furthering research and implementation of strategies to improve the care of indigenous populations with neurological and psychiatric disorders.

Educational Initiatives: Groups of students, medical residents, and faculty members from the foreign institutions traveled to Jujuy to participate in the research, learn about the province's primary health care system, and lecture on their specialty areas. Conversely, the local psychiatrists from Jujuy have participated in international meetings in the United States, the United Kingdom, Peru, Paraguay, and Bolivia. A very important landmark in capacity development for the indigenous communities of the Americas was the funding and implementation of the first international masters of science degree in clinical translational neurosciences, which was entirely focused on trainees from minority communities (NEUFIN) with cooperation from all of the institutions mentioned above and was funded by the National Institute of Mental Health and the Fogarty International Center of the United States. The first cohort of students graduated in 2017, and the second in 2019.

OUTCOMES FROM THE INTERVENTION

In terms of health outcomes, the most notable impact of implementing a system of detection, referral, and follow-up for persons with severe mental disorders was the reduction of the duration of untreated psychosis (DUP) over the course of the IMAGES study.[5] DUP can be defined as the time between the age of onset of the first psychotic symptoms or the age of first recognition of the illness, and the age at which treatment began. The importance of this measure is that DUP is a modifiable risk factor for poor health and functional outcomes and may serve as a proxy for access to mental health care. The average DUP steadily declined in consecutive years following the implementation of our training strategy, from 76.5 ± 63.3 weeks in year 1, to 11.7 ± 12.3 weeks in year 6 and above. This impressive result highlights the value of this research strategy for improving the local health care system through enhancing capacity building for all levels of care. Other tangible gains included increased and improved communications within the network, improved precision in data collection, increased systematization and time devoted to the task of detection, and referral and management of severe mental health problems.

CONCLUSIONS

International cooperation focused on innovation in the Central Andes of South America has produced unique research, educational, and healthcare opportunities as well as a set of impressive outcomes. The work done in these regions has also had a significant impact on the local communities.

The unique characteristics of a population previously unexposed to psychiatric interventions, allowed us to make observations on the natural history of schizophrenia and provided insights into the neuropsychological components of the syndrome independently from pharmacological interventions. This has led to several major scientific publications in peer-reviewed international journals.[6,18-22]

In addition, we developed a set of well-validated, culturally adapted neuropsychiatry assessment tools in the Kechwa language, as well as a neuropsychological assessment battery for intercultural, multilingual studies.

The IMAGES project has also resulted in a significant increase of the research capacity for the Province of Jujuy, thanks to sustained mentoring relationships and the resulting educational opportunities for local students and professionals.

Finally, the positive results of the task-shifting intervention and the embedding of mental health in the training of primary health workers significantly influenced local policies and primary care practice in the region.

REFERENCE LIST

1. Alvarado CA, Davee RL. Reports on the malaria eradication programs in the Americas. 11th plenary session of the Pan American Sanitary Organization meeting; 1955.
2. Alvarado, CA. Por la formación de una conciencia sanitaria en el país. Tucumán, Argentina; 1938.
3. Alvarado CA. Pautas para una cobertura sanitaria de las poblaciones rurales en medicina sanitaria y administracion de salud. Tomo II. Buenos Aires: El Ateneo; 1978.
4. World Health Organization. Atencion Primaria de Salud, Alma-Ata, Organizacion Mundial de La Salud. Geneva, Switzerland: OMS; 1978.
5. *World Health Organization. Task Shifting: Rational Redistribution of Tasks among Health Workforce Teams: Global Recommendations and Guidelines*. Geneva: World Health Organization; 2008. http://www.who.int/healthsystems/task_shifting/en/. Accessed April 11, 2018.
6. Padilla E, Molina J, Kamis D, et al. The efficacy of targeted health agent's education to reduce the duration of untreated psychosis in a rural population. *Schizophr Res.* 2015;161(2-3):184-187. doi:10.1016/j.schres.2014.10.039.
7. Wing JK, Babor T, Brugha T, et al. SCAN: Schedules for Clinical Assessment in Neuropsychiatry. *Arch Gen Psychiatry.* 1990;47(6):589-593. doi:10.1001/archpsyc.1990.01810180089012.
8. Bertelesen A, Vázquez-Barquero JL, Brugha TS. Schedules for Clinical Assessment in Neuropsychiatry 2.1 (Spanish version). World Health Organization; 1994.
9. Leff J, Sartorius N, Jablensky A, et al. The International Pilot Study of Schizophrenia: Five-year follow-up findings. *Psychological Medicine.* 1992;22:131-145.
10. Ramaker C, Marinus J, Stiggelbout AM, et al. Systematic evaluation of rating scales for impairment and disability in Parkinson's disease. *Movement Disorders.* 2002;17(5):867-876.

11. Huntington Study Group. United Huntington Disease Rating Scale: Reliability and consistency. *Movement Disorders*. 1996;11(2):136–142.

12. Cloninger CR. *The Temperament and Character Inventory (TCI): A Guide to Its Development and Use*. St. Louis: Center for Psychobiology of Personality, Washington University; 1994.

13. Sedó MA. "5 digit test": A multilingual non-reading alternative to the Stroop test. *Rev Neurol*. 2004;38(9):824–828.

14. Valdizán H. La alienación mental entre los primitivos peruanos. Doctoral thesis, Universidad Nacional Mayor de San Marcos, Facultad de Medicina; 1915. http://sisbib.unmsm.edu.pe/BibVirtual/Tesis/Antiguos/Valdizan_H_1915/indice.htm.

15. Uscamayta MJ, Sanchez Garrafa R, Escobar JI, de Erausquin G. The concept of mania in traditional Andean culture. *American Journal of Psychiatry*. May 1, 2019;176(5): 338–340.

16. Sánchez Garrafa R. *Apus de los cuatro Suyus: La construcción del mundo en el ciclo de los dioses montaña*. Lima: IEP/CBC; 2014.

17. Elferink JG. Mental disorder among the Incas in ancient Peru. *Hist Psychiatry*. 1999;10:303–310.

18. González Alemán G. Descripción y cuantificación del endofenotipo cognitivo en una población indígena con ezquizofrenia virgen de tratamiento, y demostración de la esquizotaxia en los hermanos sanos. Doctoral Dissertation. Facultad de Medicina, Universidad de Buenos Aires; 2006. http://bibliomedicinadigital.fmed.uba.ar/medicina/cgi-bin/library.cgi?a=d&c=catalogo&d=CatalogoTesis_00053.

19. Molina JL, Calvó M, Padilla E, et al. Parkinsonian motor impairment predicts personality domains related to genetic risk and treatment outcomes in schizophrenia. *NPJ Schizophr*. 2017;3:16036.

20. Molina JL, González Alemán G, Florenzano N, et al. Prediction of neurocognitive deficits by Parkinsonian motor impairment in schizophrenia: A study in neuroleptic-naïve subjects, unaffected first-degree relatives, and healthy controls from an indigenous population. *Schizophr Bull*. 2016;42(6):1486–1495.

21. Kamis D, Stratton L, Calvó M, et al. Sex and laterality differences in Parkinsonian impairment and transcranial ultrasound in never-treated schizophrenics and their first-degree relatives in an Andean population. *Schizophr Res*. 2015;164(1–3):250–255. doi:10.1016/j.schres.2015.01.035.

22. Balda M, Calvó M, Padilla E, et al. Detection, assessment, and management of schizophrenia in an Andean population of South America: Parkinsonism testing and transcranial ultrasound as preventive tools. *Focus (Am Psychiatr Publ)*. 2015;13(4): 432–440. doi:10.1176/appi.focus.20150018.

5 · GENETIC RESEARCH ON CHRONIC, SEVERE MENTAL DISORDERS IN THE PAISA POPULATION IN LATIN AMERICA

A Review of Past and Current Research

CARRIE E. BEARDEN, CARLOS LOPEZ
JARAMILLO, AND JAVIER I. ESCOBAR

The Paisa population predominates in mountainous regions of northwestern Colombia. In Colombia, *paisa* refers to people born in a relatively large geographical region of the country that includes the *departamentos* (states) of Antioquia, Caldas, Quindio, Risaralda, and at least a portion of departamento del Valle del Cauca). The original residents of the Paisa territory were Indian tribes such as the Catios, Nutabaes, Cunas, Tahamies, Quimbayas, and Emberas, who were all part of a linguistic group generically called "Caribe" by anthropologists.

During the sixteenth and seventeenth centuries, most of these natives disappeared as a consequence of either the violent actions of the European conquistadores, the epidemic illnesses they brought, or self-immolation as a reaction to the mistreatment and humiliation to which they were subjected as part of colonialism.

Gradually, the territory was filled with new immigrants, a majority of them in search of the legendary "El Dorado." The Spanish conquistador Jorge Robledo was apparently the first European to step on Paisa soil, and he established the first two Paisa towns—Cartago and Santa Fe de Antioquia—in 1540 and 1541, respectively. The first immigrants came from the Spanish regions of Extremadura and Andalucía in the sixteenth and seventeenth centuries. It is often mentioned that some of these new immigrants may have been of Jewish origin (*judios marranos*) and forced to migrate, or Jews who had converted to Catholicism during the time of the Spanish Inquisition.

The next wave of immigrants to the region arrived during the seventeenth and eighteenth centuries. These were also Spanish immigrants, although these came mainly from the Basque region. Unlike the original *conquistadores*, who generally came alone, the Basques went to the Paisa region to settle with their families. They located around the geographical region called the Aburra Valley, where the city of Medellin is located, as well as in neighboring towns such as Marinilla, El Retiro, and Santuario.

The fact that the region was quite mountainous made access into it or out of it quite difficult and isolated its residents from the rest of the country until the end of the nineteenth century. Later on, the original Paisas began migrating to the south of the Aburra Valley, starting with the old Caldas region and then moving into the more fertile plains of the Cauca River, in what is called today the coffee region of the country. In the nineteenth century, the industrialization of the region began, stimulated by the financial gains from the coffee industry; the Paisa region thus became the industrial center of the country.

The Paisa currently number about eight million people and make up about one-fifth of the population of Colombia. This population has a history of rapid expansion during ten to twenty generations, having started from a relatively small number of founders (i.e., a recent founding bottleneck.[1-4] In population genetics, the "founder effect" refers to the loss of genetic variation that occurs when a new population is established by a very small number of individuals from a larger population. Ernst Mayr first outlined this phenomenon of the founder effect in 1942 using existing theoretical work from other investigators, such as Sewall Wright.

RELEVANCE OF THE PAISA POPULATION
FOR GENETIC RESEARCH IN THE NEUROSCIENCES

Population isolates with the type of history and configuration as those seen in the Paisa region of Colombia have proven advantageous for identifying genetic variants with a high impact on disease phenotypes. Based on population genetics theory, the prediction is that bottlenecks will result in a subset of variants (including some that are deleterious) that are maintained at a much higher frequency than in outbred populations. Finland is a well-known example of this bottleneck phenomenon.[5-7] In particular, based on this history we would expect the following to be true: (1) Most common loci identified in genome-wide association studies (GWAS) will replicate in the Paisa, given its predominant European ancestry. Thus, the most common single nucleotide polymorphisms (SNPs) previously identified by GWAS can also be replicated in the Paisa population, as has been observed in the case of several complex medical disorders.[8] (2) Some ethnic-specific loci may also be observed, which will be shared with other Hispanic populations and thus are likely to have an important impact in U.S. Hispanic samples, as is the case for a newly discovered locus protective against breast cancer.[9] (3) As in other isolates, some variants will be essentially private to the Paisa[10] and thus could be identified via whole genome sequencing. (4) The genetic and cultural homogeneity of the Paisa may reduce the effects of confounders in genetic analyses.[10]

Even within Colombia, the Paisa population has unique genetic, cultural, geographical, and religious characteristics when compared to populations from other areas of the country. It exhibits high levels of endogamy and very large family networks. The traits and habits of the Paisa show they are quite attached to their native land and appear to be very conservative and religious. Genetically isolated populations like the Paisa generally have a low degree of admixture. Their genetic, cultural, and historical features, combined with their geographical location and relative geographical isolation have determined low random fluctuations in their allelic frequency that are transmitted from generation to generation.[11]

Individuals from isolate populations such as the Paisa share specific genomic regions from founder ancestors, showing such features as high levels of inbreeding and low genetic drift, which affect their genotypic composition.[12] All of these characteristics make these populations quite useful and relevant for genetic investigations of complex medical disorders.

Population genetic studies have shown that the Paisa population that inhabits the central and western branches of the Andean mountains of Colombia was formed in the 1500s mainly from the admixture of indigenous females (Amerindian women) and Spanish males primarily from the south of Spain.[13] These studies have also shown that in these populations, the Y chromosome lineage is composed of 94 percent European, 5 percent African, and 1 percent Amerindian elements, while mitochondrial DNA lineage is 90 percent Amerindian, 8 percent African, and 2 percent European.[4]

Genetic studies in the Paisa population are facilitated because residents of this region can be easily tracked and catalogued through eliciting a set of specific last names that have been shown to predict a rather homogeneous genetic makeup. This added to the environmental homogeneity may help increase the power of genetic association studies and may help to detect common and rare genetic variation underpinning different traits, phenotypes, or diseases.

James J. Parsons, a geographer from the University of California, Berkeley, pioneered studies on the Paisa population starting in the 1940s. His book *Antioqueño Colonization in Western Colombia*[14] offers a unique perspective on the Paisa population from the perspective of history, geography, and economics, and it is a frequently quoted source for studies in this population.

In this chapter, we will review findings from genetic studies of serious mental illness in the Paisa and closely related populations in Latin America. Many of these studies have taken a family-based approach, given the large well-characterized pedigrees in the region that have been essential for gene discovery in Mendelian disorders.[15,16] More recent, ongoing studies take advantage of an outstanding system of electronic health records in the state of Caldas for ascertainment of cases across diagnostic categories, as discussed in the following section.

ALZHEIMER'S DISEASE

Due to many potential advantages for genetic research, the Paisa population has been the focus of important studies in the last decades for both monogenic and polygenic diseases. One of the most relevant projects has focused on Alzheimer's Disease (AD). This research has shown that the Paisa region of Antioquia has a strong founder effect for an autosomal dominant mutation that causes early onset of AD. These studies have been led by Francisco Lopera, a neurologist from Universidad de Antioquia and also include an international consortium of investigators, mainly from the United States.

In detailed and laborious clinical and pedigree studies, Lopera first tracked this early onset dementia to several large family networks residing in Antioquia, in the middle of the Paisa region. Specific genetic studies then identified a mutation known as "E280A mutation" or "Paisa mutation" that consists of a substitution of alanine for glutamic acid in codon 280 of the presenilin 1 gene located in chromosome 14—the cause of the disease in this population of Antioquia.[17] This has created a solid clinical and genetic base for mainstream scientific research on Alzheimer's disease during the last two decades and has led to establishing strong collaborative alliances with local and international institutions to perform clinical and basic studies in the neurosciences.

One of these studies is the Alzheimer's Prevention Initiative, a prospective study funded by the National Institutes of Health (NIH), Genentech, and several foundations. This study on genetically predisposed healthy individuals has recruited 300 individuals (200 gene carriers and 100 controls) for a five-year follow-up that includes a randomized, placebo-controlled trial with crenezumab, an agent that prevents amyloid formation in the brain. The outcomes being assessed include the effects of the intervention on clinical and laboratory AD biomarkers.

COLLABORATIVE PSYCHIATRIC GENETIC STUDIES ON THE PAISA POPULATION

In the case of major mental disorders such as bipolar disorder (which has a prevalence of around 6 percent in this population), several studies have examined different components of the bipolar phenotype in efforts to gain more knowledge on the mechanisms that underlie these complex disorders. These studies have focused on the areas of neuroimaging, neuropsychology, and genetics and may contribute to establishing more stable endophenotypes to increase the precision of diagnosis and the specificity of interventions for bipolar I disorders.

The systematic study, recruitment, and assessment of hundreds of members from multigenerational and extended families of the Paisa population has clearly played a key role in the study and understanding of the genetic and biological basis of several complex disorders. This has been achieved largely due to major international collaborations and team-building aspects with international institutions such as the University of California, Los Angeles (UCLA), and Rutgers University's Robert Wood Johnson Medical School that include interdisciplinary groups (clinical psychiatrists, geneticists, mathematicians, neuroscientists, biomedical engineers, psychologist, and neuropsychologists, among others) that are all actively engaged in the process of approaching—in a well-coordinated and integrated fashion—the study of several of these disabling and complex diseases.

An international collaboration with the Grupo de Investigación en Psiquiatría (GIPSI) at Universidad de Antioquia (UdeA), led by Carlos Lopez-Jaramillo, on psychiatric genetic studies of the Paisa was initiated the late 1990s. The group has developed protocols for diagnostic interviewing, neurocognitive assessments, genealogy, and biological sample processing. GIPSI has significantly contributed to psychiatric genetics broadly. This work has included translating into Spanish the Diagnostic Interview for Genetic Studies (DIGS),[18] an instrument that has been made available to investigators via the NIMH Human Genetics Initiative. This collaboration between GIPSI and several international colleagues has led to important findings in the area of human genetics, for nonpsychiatric conditions[1,13,19,20] and specifically, for psychiatric genetics, as reviewed in detail in this chapter.[21-27] Large, extended pedigrees offer the most powerful cohorts for mapping quantitative trait loci (QTL) underlying disease-associated endophenotypes[28]; further, pedigrees in population isolates may be particularly powerful for mapping disease-associated QTL, as they should show less etiological heterogeneity than pedigrees in outbred populations.[11] These strategies informed our family-based studies of bipolar disorder, discussed in the next section.

Family Studies of Bipolar Disorder on the Paisa Population

Bipolar disorder (BP) is highly heritable,[29-32] supporting its investigation in family-based studies. However, progress in identifying disease-associated variants has been slow; variability in the definition and assessment of the affected phenotype and heterogeneity of study samples are two factors that may contribute to these difficulties.[33,34] Our initial studies of BP in the Paisa population focused on categorical disease diagnosis of severe BPI, a diagnosis requiring at least one episode of full mania, which represents the most severe and heritable form of mood disorder.[35] By studying patients with a narrowly defined phenotype, ascertained from closely related population isolates, and characterized with standardized protocols, the etiological heterogeneity of the study sample can be reduced.[36] In 2006 Herzberg and colleagues[22] conducted a whole genome linkage scan for BPI in six extended multiplex pedigrees from Antioquia, which implicated markers on 5q31–34. Notably, this was the same region highlighted in a previous genome scan of pedigrees from the Central Valley of Costa Rica (CVCR), a region with a similar demographic history and closely genetically related population.[1] This concordant signal was then followed up by genotyping additional microsatellite markers in an expanded set of pedigrees from Antioquia and the CVCR. In this combined sample, genome-wide significant linkage was found for markers in the 5q31–34 region. Notably, the linkage peak observed in these BP families shows strong overlap with regions linked in previous studies to schizophrenia or to psychosis spectrum disorders.[37] Given the focus of the studies on individuals with BPI, most of whom have experienced at least one episode of psychosis during the course of their illness, these results provide further support for the hypothesis that a locus on 5q may predispose to psychosis rather than to bipolar disorder or schizophrenia per se. However, extended analyses, including nine additional Antioquian families, did not find further linkage support for the 5q31–34 region. Several other suggestive findings were reported, including a region on chromosome 7p21.1–p22.2 previously implicated in BP in pedigrees from the Portuguese islands,[38] which is notable since both populations share ancestral contributions from the Iberian Peninsula. These results highlight the need for replication studies and meta-analyses in order to evaluate the true significance of linkage findings, given that most individual studies are likely to not be sufficiently powered to detect susceptibility loci for psychiatric disease on their own. Results from individual studies often do not coincide with most robust signals in meta-analyses, suggesting that these results may reflect larger genetic contributions of importance only to a specific population.

Intermediate Traits and the Biology of Bipolar Disorder

So far, genome-wide association studies (GWAS) have identified a handful of replicated genetic risk variants for bipolar disorder, providing clues into its genetic architecture;[39-41] however, the biology underlying the disorder remains poorly understood. The heterogeneity of BP clinical phenotypes and the commonalities between BP and other disorders in both symptomatology and genetic risk profiles support the utility of considering psychopathology dimensionally (in relation to a set of key behavioral and neurobiological domains) rather than categorically. The NIMH has established the Research Domain Criteria (RDoC) project to stimulate the adoption of a quantitative dimensional approach throughout all levels of psychiatric research.[42-44] This development has coincided with increased interest in the field in tackling the heterogeneity of psychiatric syndromes by delineating and genetically investigating endophenotypes, quantitative traits (i.e., dimensional measures) hypothesized to be components of the syndromes.

Initially the term *endophenotype* was used to describe specific insect populations[45]—in particular, that internal, not directly observable, phenotypes represent an intermediate link in a causal chain between genes and traits that can be directly observed in the field. In the subsequent application of this concept to psychiatric genetics, categorical disease phenotypes can be considered analogous to the directly observable insect traits.[46-48]

Initially, the rationale for applying the endophenotype concept to psychiatric genetic investigations is that phenotypes that are intermediate in a causal chain between gene and disease phenotypes may have a simpler genetic basis and therefore be more amenable to genetic mapping than the disease phenotypes.[39] Although more recent studies have called this assumption into question, endophenotypes unquestionably provide an opportunity to acquire a broad range of measures within and across physiological levels (i.e., brain and behavior) to characterize the underlying neurobiology of complex traits and to exploit the common genetic architecture underlying multiple phenotypes.[49] This strategy may improve the power of gene-mapping studies.

The endophenotype concept may be particularly useful for complex psychiatric disorders such as BP. BP and other serious mental illnesses (SMI) encompass a broad range of phenotypic features; however, most etiological research has focused on the overall diagnostic category rather than on its component traits. Although GWAS have recently identified the first replicated risk loci for BP,[40,41,50] the small relative increase in risk attributed to these variants likely reflects the complex genetic nature of the disorder. As such, our studies are motivated by efforts to identify heritable BP-associated quantitative traits that may offer increased power for analysis and for which higher impact variants may be detected.[40,46,51,52]

Our collaborative project, "Bipolar Endophenotypes in Population Iso-lates," investigated extended pedigrees ascertained for multiple cases of severe BP (BP-I) to delineate and genetically map quantitative traits that constituted candidate BP-I endophenotypes. Specifically, we conducted extensive phe-notyping and analysis in twenty-six pedigrees selected for multiple cases of severe BP (BP-I), using quantitative traits hypothesized to represent com-ponents of the biology underlying BP. Previous studies of these measures demonstrated an association of BP, with certain deficits, even in the case of euthymic individuals with BP diagnoses. Unaffected relatives in families with bipolar disorder were found to be intermediate between those with diagnosed BP disorder and control subjects. These phenotypes assay mul-tiple components of temperament—including impulsivity, cyclothymic temperament and perceptual creativity, and neurocognitive function and neuroanatomy—as assessed via structural magnetic resonance imaging (sMRI) and diffusion tensor imaging (DTI).

Familial aggregation of traits was assessed using SOLAR,[53] which imple-ments a variance component method to estimate the proportion of pheno-typic variance due to additive genetic factors (narrow sense heritability). This model partitions total variability into polygenic and environmental compo-nents. What we found was that of the hundreds of traits examined, the vast majority (75 percent) were significantly heritable, and about one-third were significantly associated with BP-I. About one-quarter of the traits were both heritable and associated with BP-I; these traits in particular are prioritized as the most promising phenotypes for identifying loci contributing to dis-ease risk. This group of "priority" phenotypes included some temperament traits (delusion-proneness, as measured by the Peters Delusion Inventory, and perceptual creativity, as assessed by the Barron Welsh Art Scale), some cognitive traits (verbal working memory, attentional interference, processing speed), and a large number of neuroimaging phenotypes (cortical thickness in multiple frontal regions, including the inferior frontal gyrus, thickness of the superior temporal gyrus, and corpus callosum volume. Notably, some phenotypes in this group, such as delusion-proneness,[54] appear broadly char-acteristic of the major psychoses, whereas others, such as perceptual cre-ativity, appear specific to BP predisposition.[55] Individuals diagnosed with BP are overrepresented in creative occupations compared to individuals diag-nosed with other psychiatric disorders, or to the general population.[55,56] Regarding the pattern of neuroimaging traits, these findings offer the first evidence in families of BP-related neuroanatomic alterations previously observed in case-control studies.[57,58] Broadly, we found cortical thinning in two prefrontal systems known to be involved in BP pathogenesis: (1) a cortico-cognitive system involving the lateral prefrontal cortex and all subdivisions of the inferior frontal gyrus, a brain structure implicated in attention, working memory, and inhibitory control; and (2) a ventral-limbic system associated with emotional reactivity, involving the hippocampus, amygdala and orbitofrontal cortex. Further, corpus callosum volume reduction is consistent with twin studies that have found genetically influenced alterations of this structure in BP.[59] It is also important to highlight that the profile of brain and behavioral traits affected in these unique families is similar to those identified previously in case-control samples in outbred (European and U.S.) populations. We therefore would expect that while some genetic variants contributing to these phenotypes and to risk for BP may be unique to the Paisa population, they could suggest genes or biological pathways associated with disease risk in other populations.

As a naturalistic cross-sectional study, of course, this study had limitations. In particular, psychotropic medications likely affect neuroanatomic measures in ways that are difficult to characterize in naturalistic studies, given nonrandom ascertainment to treatment and highly varying lengths of treatment and dosages.[60,61] Nevertheless, obtaining these measures in clinically unaffected family members of patients with BP is informative regarding neuroanatomic markers that index the genetic risk for the illness. Prospective longitudinal studies are also critical for answering questions regarding state versus trait anomalies.

Circadian Traits

Abnormalities in sleep and circadian rhythms are central features of BP and often persist in between episodes. Such disturbances in activity typically precede and may precipitate the initial onset of BP.[62,63] Extreme diurnal variation in mood is a prominent feature of both mania and depression, whereas shifts in circadian phase (i.e., the time within the daily activity cycle at which one typically goes to bed or awakens) can induce mania and/or reduce depression symptoms.[64]

The introduction of actigraphy (i.e., activity measurement using wristworn accelerometers) as a research tool has permitted the initiation of large-scale investigation of sleep and circadian rhythm traits as components of BP, but few conclusive findings have emerged from such research. In the first genetic investigation of a comprehensive set of sleep and circadian measures in humans, we recorded activity in 136 euthymic BP-I individuals and 422 of their non–BP-I relatives from the pedigrees described above, for an average of two weeks. For each actigraphy phenotype, we evaluated association with BP-I and assessed its heritability and then performed genome-wide genetic linkage analyses on all significantly heritable traits.

Findings indicated substantial genetic influence on sleep and activity traits, with 67 percent of phenotypes investigated showing significant heritability. Further, there was a consistent set of findings for phenotypes significantly associated with BP-I; overall activity was lower in euthymic BP-I individuals than in their non–BP-I relatives, reflecting a longer sleep duration and a later awakening time, meaning a shorter duration of the active phase. Furthermore, during the active phase, BP-I individuals had fewer total minutes scored as awake and more variability in total minutes asleep. BP-I individuals also had lower amplitude, mainly due to lower activity levels during the least active hours of the day. In order to uncover genetic loci with the largest impact on sleep and activity phenotypes in these families, we conducted genome-wide linkage analysis using a dense set of SNPs. Our primary analyses focused on thirteen phenotypes that we considered most relevant to BP. The strongest linkage was for the rest-activity phenotype "interdaily stability," which represents the variability of activity level on an hourly basis. For this phenotype, we observed a maximum logarithm (base 10) of odds (LOD) score of 4.73, near chromosome 12pter. This exceeds the traditional genome-wide significance threshold of $p < 10^{-4}$ and remained significant after correcting for the thirteen phenotypes tested. In the same region of linkage to interdaily stability, we observed suggestive linkage for two additional phenotypes, the mean number of sleep bouts in the awake period, and amplitude (the difference in activity between the five most active hours and the ten least active hours), with peak LOD scores of 2.53 and 2.13, respectively. Interdaily stability and mean number of sleep bouts showed a strongly negative genetic correlation ($rho_g = -.93$), and joint multipoint linkage analysis suggested complete pleiotropy, indicating a common genetic component to both phenotypes. Additionally, interdaily stability showed a strong (positive) genetic correlation ($rho_g = 0.92$) with amplitude; their joint linkage analysis ($LOD = 3.41$) suggests near-complete pleiotropy between these phenotypes. This highlights the importance of this genomic region for the regulation of aspects of circadian activity. Several genes in this region may influence activity-related behaviors, including the histone lysine demethylase *JARID1a* (*KMD5A*) and calcium channel subunit 1C (*CACNA1C*). *JARID1a* forms a complex with the core clock proteins BMAL1 and CLOCK. In mammalian cells, depletion of JARID1a has been shown to shorten the circadian period.[65] Notably, *CACNA1C* has shown genome-wide significant association to BP, as well as other psychiatric disorders, in multiple GWA studies.[66,67] There is also evidence for a role of this gene in insomnia and sleep habits.[68] Whole-genome sequencing studies, now underway in these pedigrees, will allow evaluation of variants in the genes discussed above in relation to sleep and activity phenotypes, as well as other genes in this region.

Genome-wide Gene Expression

We also assessed the heritability and genetic regulation of gene expression in lymphoblastoid cell lines (LCL) in these families. Given increasing evidence that a substantial proportion of local genetic regulation is conserved across tissues,[69] we used LCLs to estimate heritability, evaluate the relative contributions of local versus distal genomic variation, identify variants with regulatory effects, and analyze the role of multiple associated SNPs in the same region. The pedigree design allowed us to compare estimates of the heritability of gene expression obtained using both traditional and genotype-based methods. We investigated the architecture of genetic regulation, including the extent to which gene expression is influenced by local versus distal variants on the genome and how many variants affect the expression of a given gene.[70] Findings indicated that variation in expression values is heritable, with 18 percent of probes showing heritability > 0.2; moreover, in this related sample, theoretical kinship coefficients and genotype correlations for estimation of heritability yielded similar results. In addition, we identified genetic variants, which regulate gene expression and are potential candidates for future studies to establish the genetic basis of complex traits related to serious mental illness. As such, these findings provide insight into the architecture of genetic regulation in this unique Latin American study population.

In summary, the work from this study represents the most comprehensive evaluation to date of BP component phenotypes; in it we delineated measures that may help elucidate the genetic contribution to BP-I risk. It demonstrated the heritability and association with BP-I of > 100 neurocognitive, temperament, and structural MRI phenotypes[25,26] and provided the first delineation and genetic analysis of BP-I related to circadian phenotypes.[27] Ongoing studies in these pedigrees include whole genome sequencing (WGS) analyses of BP-I and heritable quantitative traits.

WGS studies of pedigrees in founder populations, such as the Paisa, offer four advantages for identifying variants with a large phenotypic impact. First, in population isolates, rapid expansion from a bottleneck has, by genetic drift, dramatically increased the frequency of some rare deleterious variants.[25,71,72] This process facilitates the identification across families of variants with a large phenotypic effect on the disease or endophenotypes; these variants can then be analyzed through imputation in much larger genotyped samples. While such variants may be limited to the population isolates in which they are identified, they serve to prioritize specific genes (or other functional elements) for investigation in large samples. Second, the pedigree structure permits cost-effective implementation of WGS; by sequencing selected family members, one can impute the sequence of their genotyped relatives. Third, in pedigree data, it is more straightforward to distinguish true variants from sequencing artifacts, and transmitted alleles from *de novo* mutations.[73] Finally, the clustering of common disorders in pedigrees is a signpost for the presence of large-effect variants;[74] if pedigrees are sufficiently large, it may be possible to observe segregation between phenotypes and variants across several generations. For example, variants that co-segregate with both substance-use disorders and mood disorder can illuminate the biological underpinnings of comorbidity.

Motivation to Develop New Project: Genetics of Transdiagnostic Serious Mental Illness

Historically, Emil Kraepelin and colleagues divided serious mental illness (SMI) into two distinct categories: psychotic disorders (the schizophrenia spectrum; SCZ) and mood disorders (the BP spectrum, incorporating BP and major depressive disorder), a dichotomy that has lasted for over a century.[75-78] Among mental disorders, these categories are the largest contributors to global disease burden.[79] However, growing evidence that these categories have common genetic underpinnings,[66,80] together with the pattern of overlapping symptoms between them, has led to increasing calls to abandon this dichotomy. As noted earlier, the NIH RDoC initiative aims to link specific behavioral constructs to hypothesized underlying neural circuitry by adopting classification systems based on dimensional domains.

While this is an important effort, the current classification system of SMI has value in that it (1) reflects differences between categories in disease trajectory and prognosis that have been observed consistently and that provide important information for patients and their families; (2) recognizes clinically meaningful treatment outcomes that are distinctive to particular diagnoses (e.g., the switch to mania that often occurs when BP-affected individuals receive antidepressant drugs[81]); and (3) forms the basis for health statistics around the world.[82-84] To simply abandon this dichotomy would transform virtually all levels of mental health research and practice, while empirical evidence for the biological validity of alternative frameworks, such as RDoC, remains sparse. It is therefore critical that we establish a stronger scientific foundation on which to base new classification systems for SMI.

Psychiatric geneticists focused for more than two decades on efforts to identify single major loci contributing to risk for SMI disorders,[85] and the field largely disregarded models predicting that polygenic inheritance of multiple variants, each with a small phenotypic impact, would better explain the distribution of these disorders in the population.[86] The recent large-scale GWAS of these disorders have yielded overwhelming evidence bearing out this prediction[87] and have shown that the entirety of common variation (as measured by polygenic risk scores; PRS) provides a framework for comparisons of phenotypic categories. These comparisons confirm the high degree of genetic correlation between mood and psychotic disorders.[88-91] However, the multiplicity of assessment tools employed at different sites, and between SCZ and BP datasets, may have weakened prior findings and precluded particular analyses—for example, of symptom-level data.[92] In contrast to fields such as cardiology,[93] the paucity of dimensional phenotype data in psychiatric GWAS datasets has limited our ability to make full use of GWAS data.

As such, the premise of our new study of the genetics of serious mental illness in the Paisa population is that we can use genetic analysis of common genetic variation (SNPs) to help establish a biologically valid nosology for SMI, but we need different kinds of datasets than we have now. With symptom-level and quantitative trait data in SMI-affected individuals uniformly ascertained across diagnostic categories, we may identify genetic relationships stronger than those observed for the diagnoses themselves. There are three lines of evidence that support this premise: First, SMI categories are significantly genetically correlated, evidenced through significantly associated loci and through PRS.[88] Second, symptoms that occur across the

SMI dichotomy are clinically important and biologically valid, independent of the syndromal diagnoses to which these symptoms contribute—for example, suicidal ideation is a core symptom of mood disorders that is also common across the SCZ spectrum,[94] and psychotic symptoms, which are core to SCZ, are common in both BP and MDD.[95] Third, quantitative trait measures across domains are heritable and meaningfully related to SMI—for example, several studies have shown a genetic relationship between SCZ and measures of cognitive function.[96]

This project has the goal to ascertain a prospective sample of 8,000 individuals who carry an SMI diagnosis (across the broad spectra of mood and psychotic disorders), drawn from the Paisa ethnic population from a single hospital in northwestern Colombia. We are obtaining both extensive phenotype data and genome-wide genotype data from these individuals along with 2,000 sex- and age-matched controls from the same population. Analyzing these data will advance our understanding of the genetic underpinnings of SMI by identifying the relationship between common genetic variations and particular phenotypic measures that have not previously been investigated in a large, uniformly assessed sample. Specifically, we plan to (1) evaluate the relationship between genome-wide significant variants from ongoing international meta-analyses of SMI diagnoses (SCZ, BP, and MDD[97-102]) and specific symptoms of SMI (across diagnoses); (2) analyze the relationship between PRS and SMI at the level of diagnoses, specific symptoms, and quantitative traits that may index core deficits in SMI; and (3) estimate the heritability of the quantitative traits and perform association analyses of the heritable traits. This project avoids pitfalls of prior studies focused on specific diagnostic categories by employing a standard set of measures across diagnoses and a uniform method of ascertainment via electronic medical record data (EMR).

Two factors motivated us to expand our efforts from Antioquia to Caldas: First, the research team in Colombia developed a uniquely valuable resource for psychiatric research, using the EMR to recruit patients with SMI across diagnostic categories. Second, analyses of samples from representative populations in each state suggest that there are no substantial genetic differences between them, and that the Caldas population descends mainly from Antioquian families.[3] To our knowledge, this will be the first large-scale study to evaluate the comparative validity of dimensional to categorical systems for classification of major psychiatric disorders, employing PRS as indices of validity and using rigorously and uniformly collected symptom-level data across the SMI diagnostic categories (psychotic and mood disorders).

Other Examples of Founder Effects in Colombia

In addition to the Paisa, there are other populations in Colombia that have unique genetic backgrounds. For example, in the district of Ricaurte, west of Bogota, there is a high proportion of intellectual disability. Population screening of the entire town (1,186 inhabitants in 2018)[103] revealed a disproportionately high prevalence of carriers of the FMR1 expanded allele (premutations and full mutations), which causes Fragile X syndrome (FXS), the most common cause of inherited intellectual disability and autism. Carrier frequency of the full mutation allele was 343 times higher among males in Ricaurte and 226 times higher among females compared to expected population prevalence rates. This is among the highest carrier frequencies ever reported, suggesting that Ricaurte constitutes a genetic cluster of FXS. All of the expanded FMR1 alleles in the population were linked to three independent pedigrees, and most likely the expanded allele arrived with the original founders of Ricaurte.

In addition, other diseases (both Mendelian and complex disorders) are frequently found in this population. These include albinism, nonsyndromic cleft lip and palate, Parkinson's disease and dementias, and rheumatologic and autoimmune conditions, as well as other complex psychiatric disorders such as schizophrenia, major depressive disorder, and attention deficit/hyperactivity disorder.[104,105]

CONCLUSIONS

Across biomedicine, including psychiatry, large-scale GWAS have revolutionized our understanding of disease, both through the identification of thousands of replicated loci and by the use of polygenic risk scores as a method for quantifying the relationship of phenotypes with each other and with a number of variables not previously amenable to biological analyses. Large-scale exome and whole-genome sequencing studies of serious mental illness conducted over the next few years in both outbred populations and special populations such as the Paisa will provide, for the first time, the opportunity to identify low-frequency or rare variants that exert a large impact on BP and/or its endophenotypes. The results of these studies will guide a new generation of investigations into the basic biology (both shared and unique) across disorders and will inform the search for improved treatments and preventive interventions.

REFERENCE LIST

1. Service S, DeYoung J, Karayiorgou M, et al. Magnitude and distribution of linkage disequilibrium in population isolates and implications for genome-wide association studies. *Nat Genet.* 2006;38(5):556–560.

2. Carvajal-Carmona LG, Soto ID, Pineda N, et al. Strong Amerind/white sex bias and a possible Sephardic contribution among the founders of a population in northwest Colombia. *Am J Hum Genet.* 2000;67(5):1287–1295.

3. Bedoya G, Garcia J, Montoya P, et al. [Isonymy analysis between 2 populations in northwestern Colombia]. *Biomedica: Revista del Instituto Nacional de Salud.* 2006;26(4): 538–545.

4. Bedoya G, Montoya P, Garcia J, et al. Admixture dynamics in Hispanics: A shift in the nuclear genetic ancestry of a South American population isolate. *Proc Natl Acad Sci U S A.* 2006;103(19):7234–7239.

5. Stoll G, Pietilainen OP, Linder B, et al. Deletion of TOP3beta, a component of FMRP-containing mRNPs, contributes to neurodevelopmental disorders. *Nat Neurosci.* 2013;16(9):1228–1237.

6. Lim ET, Wurtz P, Havulinna AS, et al. Distribution and medical impact of loss-of-function variants in the Finnish founder population. *PLoS Genet.* 2014;10(7):e1004494.

7. Service SK, Teslovich TM, Fuchsberger C, et al. Re-sequencing expands our understanding of the phenotypic impact of variants at GWAS loci. *PLoS Genet.* 2014;10(1): e1004147.

8. Leslie EJ, Carlson JC, Shaffer JR, et al. A multi-ethnic genome-wide association study identifies novel loci for non-syndromic cleft lip with or without cleft palate on 2p24.2, 17q23, and 19q13. *Hum Mol Genet.* 2016;25(13):2862–2872.

9. Fejerman L, Ahmadiyeh N, Hu D, et al. Genome-wide association study of breast cancer in Latinas identifies novel protective variants on 6q25. *Nat Commun.* 2014;5: 5260.

10. Velez JI, Lopera F, Sepulveda-Falla D, et al. APOE*E2 allele delays age of onset in PSEN1 E280A Alzheimer's disease. *Molecular Psychiatry.* 2016. 21(7):916-24.

11. Peltonen L, Palotie A, Lange K. Use of population isolates for mapping complex traits. *Nat Rev Genet.* 2000;1(3):182–190.

12. Jobling M, Hollox E, Hurles M, Kivisild T, Tyler-Smith C. Transnational isolates. In: Jobling M et al, ed. *Human Evolutionary Genetics.* 2nd ed. New York and London: Garland Science; 2004:441–467.

13. Carvajal-Carmona L, Ophoff R, Service S, et al. Genetic demography of Antioquia (Columbia) and the Central Valley of Costa Rica. *Hum Genet.* 2003;112:534–541.

14. Parsons JJ. *Antioqueno Colonization in Western Colombia.* Rev. ed. Berkeley: University of California Press; 1968.

15. Puffenberger EG, Kauffman ER, Bolk S, et al. Identity-by-descent and association mapping of a recessive gene for Hirschsprung disease on human chromosome 13q22. *Hum Mol Genet.* 1994;3(8):1217–1225.

16. Levy-Lahad E, Wijsman EM, Nemens E, et al. A familial Alzheimer's disease locus on chromosome 1. *Science.* 1995;269(5226):970–973.

17. Lendon CL, Martinez A, Behrens IM, et al. E280A PS-1 mutation causes Alzheimer's disease but age of onset is not modified by ApoE alleles. *Hum Mutat.* 1997;10(3): 186–195.

18. Nurnberger Jr. JI, Blehar MC, Kaufmann CA, et al. Diagnostic interview for genetic studies: Rationale, unique features, and training. NIMH Genetics Initiative. *Arch Gen Psychiatry.* 1994;51(11):849–859.

19. Service S, Molina J, Deyoung J, et al. Results of a SNP genome screen in a large Costa Rican pedigree segregating for severe bipolar disorder. *Am J Med Genet B Neuropsychiatr Genet.* 2006;141(4):367–373.

20. Reich D, Patterson N, Campbell D, et al. Reconstructing Native American population history. *Nature.* 2012;488(7411):370–374.

21. Ospina-Duque J, Duque C, Carvajal-Carmona L, et al. An association study of bipolar mood disorder (type I) with the 5-HTTLPR serotonin transporter polymorphism in a human population isolate from Colombia. *Neurosci Lett.* 2000;292(3): 199–202.

22. Herzberg I, Jasinska A, Garcia J, et al. Convergent linkage evidence from two Latin-American population isolates supports the presence of a susceptibility locus for bipolar disorder in 5q31-34. *Hum Mol Genet.* 2006;15(21):3146–3153.

23. Jasinska AJ, Service S, Jawaheer D, et al. A narrow and highly significant linkage signal for severe bipolar disorder in the chromosome 5q33 region in Latin American pedigrees. *American Journal of Medical Genetics Part B, Neuropsychiatric Genetics: The Official Publication of the International Society of Psychiatric Genetics.* 2009;150B(7): 998–1006.

24. Kremeyer B, Garcia J, Muller H, et al. Genome-wide linkage scan of bipolar disorder in a Colombian population isolate replicates loci on chromosomes 7p21-22, 1p31, 16p12, and 21q21-22 and identifies a novel locus on chromosome 12q. *Hum Hered.* 2010;70(4):255–268.

25. Fears SC, Service SK, Kremeyer B, et al. Multisystem component phenotypes of bipolar disorder for genetic investigations of extended pedigrees. *JAMA Psychiatry.* 2014;71(4):375–387.

26. Fears SC, Schur R, Sjouwerman R, et al. Brain structure-function associations in multi-generational families genetically enriched for bipolar disorder. *Brain.* 2015;138(7): 2087–2102.

27. Pagani L, St Clair PA, Teshiba TM, et al. Genetic contributions to circadian activity rhythm and sleep pattern phenotypes in pedigrees segregating for severe bipolar disorder. *Proc Natl Acad Sci U S A.* 2016;113(6):E754–761.

28. Williams JT, Begleiter H, Porjesz B, et al. Joint multipoint linkage analysis of multivariate qualitative and quantitative traits. II. Alcoholism and event-related potentials. *Am J Hum Genet.* 1999;65(4):1148–1160.

29. Dick DM, Foroud T, Edenberg HJ, et al. Apparent replication of suggestive linkage on chromosome 16 in the NIMH genetics initiative bipolar pedigrees. *Am J Med Genet.* 2002;114(4):407–412.

30. Gershon ES. Bipolar illness and schizophrenia as oligogenic diseases: Implications for the future. *Biol Psychiatry.* 2000;47(3):240–244.

31. Kieseppa T, Partonen T, Haukka J, Kaprio J, Lonnqvist J. High concordance of bipolar I disorder in a nationwide sample of twins. *Am J Psychiatry.* 2004;161(10): 1814–1821.

32. McGuffin P, Rijsdijk F, Andrew M, Sham P, Katz R, Cardno A. The heritability of bipolar affective disorder and the genetic relationship to unipolar depression. *Arch Gen Psychiatry.* 2003;60(5):497–502.

33. Bearden CE, Jasinska AJ, Freimer NB. Methodological issues in molecular genetic studies of mental disorders. *Annu Rev Clin Psychol.* 2009;5:49–69.

34. Bearden CE, Reus VI, Freimer NB. Why genetic investigation of psychiatric disorders is so difficult. *Curr Opin Genet Dev.* 2004;14(3):280–286.

35. Freimer NB, Reus VI, Escamilla M, et al. An approach to investigating linkage for bipolar disorder using large Costa Rican pedigrees. *Am J Med Genet.* 1996;67(3): 254–263.

36. Ophoff RA, Escamilla MA, Service SK, et al. Genomewide linkage disequilibrium mapping of severe bipolar disorder in a population isolate. *Am J Hum Genet.* 2002;71(3): 565–574.

37. Gurling HM, Kalsi G, Brynjolfson J, et al. Genomewide genetic linkage analysis confirms the presence of susceptibility loci for schizophrenia, on chromosomes 1q32.2, 5q33.2, and 8p21-22 and provides support for linkage to schizophrenia, on chromosomes 11q23.3-24 and 20q12.1-11.23. *Am J Hum Genet.* 2001;68(3):661–673.

38. Pato CN, Pato MT, Kirby A, et al. Genome-wide scan in Portuguese Island families implicates multiple loci in bipolar disorder: Fine mapping adds support on chromosomes 6 and 11. *Am J Med Genet B Neuropsychiatr Genet.* 2004;127B(1):30–34.

39. Gottesman II, Gould TD. The endophenotype concept in psychiatry: Etymology and strategic intentions. *American Journal of Psychiatry.* 2003;160:636–645.

40. Sklar P, Smoller JW, Fan J, et al. Whole-genome association study of bipolar disorder. *Mol Psychiatry.* 2008;13(6):558–569.

41. Sullivan PF, Daly MJ, O'Donovan M. Genetic architectures of psychiatric disorders: The emerging picture and its implications. *Nat Rev Genet.* 2012;13(8):537–551.

42. Insel T, Cuthbert B, Garvey M, et al. Research domain criteria (RDoC): Toward a new classification framework for research on mental disorders. *Am J Psychiatry.* 2010;167(7):748–751.

43. Insel TR. The NIMH Research Domain Criteria (RDoC) Project: Precision medicine for psychiatry. *Am J Psychiatry.* 2014;171(4):395–397.

44. Cuthbert BN, Insel TR. Toward the future of psychiatric diagnosis: The seven pillars of RDoC. *BMC Med.* 2013;11:126.

45. John B, Lewis KR. Chromosome variability and geographic distribution in insects. *Science.* 1966;152(3723):711–721.

46. Bearden CE, Freimer NB. Endophenotypes for psychiatric disorders: Ready for primetime? *Trends Genet.* 2006;22(6):306–313.

47. Casey BJ, Craddock N, Cuthbert BN, Hyman SE, Lee FS, Ressler KJ. DSM-5 and RDoC: Progress in psychiatry research? *Nat Rev Neurosci.* 2013;14(11):810–814.

48. Gottesman, II, Shields J. Genetic theorizing and schizophrenia. *Br J Psychiatry.* 1973;122(566):15–30.

49. Flint J, Timpson N, Munafo M. Assessing the utility of intermediate phenotypes for genetic mapping of psychiatric disease. *Trends Neurosci.* 2014;37(12):733–741.

50. Ferreira MA, O'Donovan MC, Meng YA, et al. Collaborative genome-wide association analysis supports a role for ANK3 and CACNA1C in bipolar disorder. *Nat Genet.* 2008;40(9):1056–1058.

51. Kendler KS, Neale MC. Endophenotype: A conceptual analysis. *Mol Psychiatry.* 2010;15(8):789–797.

52. Walters JT, Owen MJ. Endophenotypes in psychiatric genetics. *Mol Psychiatry.* 2007;12(10):886–890.

53. Almasy L, Blangero J. Multipoint quantitative-trait linkage analysis in general pedigrees. *Am J Hum Genet.* 1998;62(5):1198–1211.

54. Schurhoff F, Szoke A, Meary A, et al. Familial aggregation of delusional proneness in schizophrenia and bipolar pedigrees. *Am J Psychiatry.* 2003;160(7):1313–1319.

55. Jamison KR. Great wits and madness: More near allied? *Br J Psychiatry.* 2011;199(5): 351–352.

56. Kyaga S, Lichtenstein P, Boman M, Hultman C, Langstrom N, Landen M. Creativity and mental disorder: Family study of 300,000 people with severe mental disorder. *Br J Psychiatry.* 2011;199(5):373–379.

57. Arnone D, Cavanagh J, Gerber D, Lawrie SM, Ebmeier KP, McIntosh AM. Magnetic resonance imaging studies in bipolar disorder and schizophrenia: Meta-analysis. *Br J Psychiatry.* 2009;195(3):194–201.

58. Hallahan B, Newell J, Soares JC, et al. Structural magnetic resonance imaging in bipolar disorder: An international collaborative mega-analysis of individual adult patient data. *Biol Psychiatry.* 2011;69(4):326–335.

59. Bearden CE, van Erp TG, Dutton RA, et al. Mapping corpus callosum morphology in twin pairs discordant for bipolar disorder. *Cereb Cortex.* 2011;21(10):2415–2424.

60. Bearden CE, Thompson PM, Dutton RA, et al. Three-dimensional mapping of hippocampal anatomy in unmedicated and lithium-treated patients with bipolar disorder. *Neuropsychopharmacology.* 2008;33(6):1229–1238.

61. Kempton MJ, Geddes JR, Ettinger U, Williams SC, Grasby PM. Meta-analysis, database, and meta-regression of 98 structural imaging studies in bipolar disorder. *Arch Gen Psychiatry.* 2008;65(9):1017–1032.

62. Jackson A, Cavanagh J, Scott J. A systematic review of manic and depressive pro-dromes. *J Affect Disord.* 2003;74(3):209–217.

63. Leibenluft E, Albert PS, Rosenthal NE, Wehr TA. Relationship between sleep and mood in patients with rapid-cycling bipolar disorder. *Psychiatry Res.* 1996;63(2–3): 161–168.

64. Benedetti F, Barbini B, Colombo C, Smeraldi E. Chronotherapeutics in a psychiatric ward. *Sleep Med Rev.* 2007;11(6):509–522.

65. DiTacchio L, Le HD, Vollmers C, et al. Histone lysine demethylase JARID1a activates CLOCK-BMAL1 and influences the circadian clock. *Science.* 2011;333(6051): 1881–1885.

66. Cross-Disorder Group of the Psychiatric Genomics Consortium, Lee SH, Ripke S, et al. Genetic relationship between five psychiatric disorders estimated from genome-wide SNPs. *Nat Genet.* 2013;45(9):984–994.

67. Ferreira MA, O'Donovan MC, Meng YA, et al. Collaborative genome-wide association analysis supports a role for ANK3 and CACNA1C in bipolar disorder. *Nat Genet.* 2008. 40(9):1056–8.

68. Parsons MJ, Lester KJ, Barclay NL, Nolan PM, Eley TC, Gregory AM. Replication of Genome-Wide Association Studies (GWAS) loci for sleep in the British G1219 cohort. *Am J Med Genet B Neuropsychiatr Genet.* 2013;162B(5):431–438.

69. Flutre T, Wen X, Pritchard J, Stephens M. A statistical framework for joint eQTL analysis in multiple tissues. *PLoS Genet.* 2013;9(5):e1003486.

70. Peterson CB, Service SK, Jasinska AJ, et al. Characterization of expression quantitative trait loci in pedigrees from Colombia and Costa Rica ascertained for bipolar disorder. *PLoS Genet.* 2016;12(5):e1006046.

71. Ripke S, O'Dushlaine C, Chambert K, et al. Genome-wide association analysis identifies 13 new risk loci for schizophrenia. *Nat Genet.* 2013;45(10):1150–1159.

72. Stull GW, Moore MJ, Mandala VS, et al. A targeted enrichment strategy for massively parallel sequencing of angiosperm plastid genomes. *Appl Plant Sci.* 2013;1(2).

73. Roach JC, Glusman G, Smit AF, et al. Analysis of genetic inheritance in a family quartet by whole-genome sequencing. *Science.* 2010;328(5978):636–639.

74. Cirulli ET, Goldstein DB. Uncovering the roles of rare variants in common disease through whole-genome sequencing. *Nat Rev Genet.* 2010;11(6):415–425.

75. Brown AS. The Kraepelinian dichotomy from the perspective of prenatal infectious and immunologic insults. *Schizophr Bull.* 2015;41(4):786–791.

76. Kotov R, Leong SH, Mojtabai R, et al. Boundaries of schizoaffective disorder: Revisiting Kraepelin. *JAMA Psychiatry.* 2013;70(12):1276–1286.

77. Kuswanto CN, Sum MY, Sim K. Neurocognitive functioning in schizophrenia and bipolar disorder: Clarifying concepts of diagnostic dichotomy vs. continuum. *Front Psychiatry.* 2013;4:162.

78. Wexler BE. Beyond the Kraepelinean dichotomy. *Biol Psychiatry.* 1992;31(6): 539–541.

79. Global Burden of Disease Study Collaborators. Global, regional, and national incidence, prevalence, and years lived with disability for 301 acute and chronic diseases and

injuries in 188 countries, 1990–2013: A systematic analysis for the Global Burden of Disease Study 2013. *Lancet.* 2015;386(9995):743–800.

80. Cross-Disorder Phenotype Group of the Psychiatric GWAS Consortium, Craddock N, Kendler K, et al. Dissecting the phenotype in genome-wide association studies of psychiatric illness. *Br J Psychiatry.* 2009;195(2):97–99.

81. Pacchiarotti I, Bond DJ, Baldessarini RJ, et al. The International Society for Bipolar Disorders (ISBD) task force report on antidepressant use in bipolar disorders. *Am J Psychiatry.* 2013;170(11):1249–1262.

82. Charlson FJ, Baxter AJ, Cheng HG, Shidhaye R, Whiteford HA. The burden of mental, neurological, and substance use disorders in China and India: A systematic analysis of community representative epidemiological studies. *Lancet.* 2016;Epub 17 May 2016.

83. Lopez AD, Murray CC. The global burden of disease, 1990–2020. *Nat Med.* 1998;4(11):1241–1243.

84. Prince M, Patel V, Saxena S, et al. No health without mental health. *Lancet.* 2007;370(9590):859–877.

85. McCarroll SA, Feng G, Hyman SE. Genome-scale neurogenetics: Methodology and meaning. *Nat Neurosci.* 2014;17(6):756-763.

86. Gottesman, II, Shields J. A critical review of recent adoption, twin, and family studies of schizophrenia: Behavioral genetics perspectives. *Schizophr Bull.* 1976;2(3): 360–401.

87. International Schizophrenia Consortium, Purcell SM, Wray NR, et al. Common polygenic variation contributes to risk of schizophrenia and bipolar disorder. *Nature.* 2009;460(7256):748–752.

88. Geschwind DH, Flint J. Genetics and genomics of psychiatric disease. *Science.* 2015;349(6255):1489–1494.

89. Laursen TM, Agerbo E, Pedersen CB. Bipolar disorder, schizoaffective disorder, and schizophrenia overlap: A new comorbidity index. *Journal of Clinical Psychiatry.* 2009;70(10):1432–1438.

90. Rosen C, Marvin R, Reilly JL, et al. Phenomenology of first-episode psychosis in schizophrenia, bipolar disorder, and unipolar depression: A comparative analysis. *Clinical Schizophrenia and Related Psychoses.* 2012;6(3):145–151.

91. Scully PJ, Owens JM, Kinsella A, Waddington JL. Schizophrenia, schizoaffective and bipolar disorder within an epidemiologically complete, homogeneous population in rural Ireland: Small area variation in rate. *Schizophrenia Research.* 2004;67(2–3): 143–155.

92. Ruderfer DM, Fanous AH, Ripke S, et al. Polygenic dissection of diagnosis and clinical dimensions of bipolar disorder and schizophrenia. *Molecular Psychiatry.* 2014;19(9): 1017–1024.

93. Ripatti P, Ramo JT, Soderlund S, et al. The contribution of GWAS loci in familial dyslipidemias. *PLoS Genet.* 2016;12(5):e1006078.

94. Majadas S, Olivares J, Galan J, Diez T. Prevalence of depression and its relationship with other clinical characteristics in a sample of patients with stable schizophrenia. *Comprehensive Psychiatry.* 2012;53(2):145–151.

95. Tamminga CA, Ivleva EI, Keshavan MS, et al. Clinical phenotypes of psychosis in the Bipolar-Schizophrenia Network on Intermediate Phenotypes (B-SNIP). *Am J Psychiatry.* 2013;170(11):1263–1274.

96. Trampush JW, Yang MLZ, Yu J, et al. GWAS meta-analysis reveals novel loci and genetic correlates for general cognitive function: A report from the COGENT consortium. *Mol Psychiatry.* 2017;22(11):1651–1652.

97. Costas J, Carrera N, Alonso P, et al. Exon-focused genome-wide association study of obsessive-compulsive disorder and shared polygenic risk with schizophrenia. *Transl Psychiatry.* 2016;6:e768.

98. Hauberg ME, Roussos P, Grove J, Borglum AD, Mattheisen M, Schizophrenia Working Group of the Psychiatric Genomics Consortium. Analyzing the role of microRNAs in schizophrenia in the context of common genetic risk variants. *JAMA Psychiatry.* 2016;73(4):369–377.

99. Hou L, Heilbronner U, Degenhardt F, et al. Genetic variants associated with response to lithium treatment in bipolar disorder: A genome-wide association study. *Lancet.* 2016;387(10023):1085–1093.

100. Hubbard L, Tansey KE, Rai D, et al. Evidence of common genetic overlap between schizophrenia and cognition. *Schizophr Bull.* 2016;42(3):832–842.

101. Schizophrenia Working Group of the Psychiatric Genomics Consortium. Biological insights from 108 schizophrenia-associated genetic loci. *Nature.* 2014;511(7510):421–427.

102. Sokolowski M, Wasserman J, Wasserman D. Polygenic associations of neurodevelopmental genes in suicide attempt. *Molecular Psychiatry.* 2016; 21(10):1381–90.

103. Saldarriaga W, Forero-Forero JV, Gonzalez-Teshima LY, et al. Genetic cluster of fragile X syndrome in a Colombian district. *J Hum Genet.* 2018;63(4):509–516.

104. Arcos-Burgos M, Jain M, Acosta MT, et al. A common variant of the latrophilin 3 gene, LPHN3, confers susceptibility to ADHD and predicts effectiveness of stimulant medication. *Mol Psychiatry.* 2010;15(11):1053–1066.

105. Arboleda-Velasquez JF, Lopera F, Lopez E, et al. C455R notch3 mutation in a Colombian CADASIL kindred with early onset of stroke. *Neurology.* 2002;59(2):277–279.

6 · A BRIEF REJOINDER AND FUTURE PROJECTIONS

JAVIER I. ESCOBAR

The information presented in this book provides a glimpse of the field of global mental health, with a particular focus on Latino and Spanish-speaking populations. It is hoped that it will stimulate further debate and discussions on how to move the field forward.

More than a thorough and systematic recounting or cataloguing of activities and progress in the global mental health field, a main goal of this book is to present a few representative or colorful vignettes in an effort to illustrate the promises of building successful collaborations that allow the performance, at distant global sites, of mainstream scientific research in the neurosciences. I have selected these, rather selfishly, on the basis of ongoing collaborations and collegial contacts. Also, potential pitfalls of the evidence-based model are hinted here and there, as well as the potential for abuse or misuse when broadly expanding mental health models and interventions to the field.

The first chapter summarized most of the existing evidence, highlighting the most pressing and unrelenting mental health problems worldwide and briefly cataloguing a growing number of evidence-based interventions that are being implemented in many regions of the globe. I hope that this chapter provided a general introduction to the chapters that followed, emphasizing existing gaps and strengths and drafting a plan of action for interventions and research, with a particular focus on Latin America and the Spanish-speaking world.

In chapter 2, a new perspective, the Culturally Infused Engagement model, grounded on important work in the United States for assessing ethnic minorities, is presented to the global mental health field, as an innovative and relevant new model for working with patients from diverse cultural backgrounds. This should complement nicely other available culturally focused approaches to mental health, such as the cultural formulation proposed by Roberto Lewis-Fernandez as part of the DSM-5, the most recent diagnostic system in North America.[61]

Chapter 3 highlighted the abuse of psychiatry globally by introducing examples from the past, including little-known historical accounts of this abuse in Latin America and, particularly, a historical account of the glaring misuse of academic psychiatry during Franco's dictatorship in Spain. The latter is particularly poignant, but several of the other examples in Latin America and even in the United States illustrated the negative potential for applying globally unrestrained theories and practices and remind us about the need to remain vigilant.

Chapters 4 and 5, focusing on specific research projects that are currently ongoing in South America, highlighted first and foremost the relevance and benefits of successful international collaborations. Indeed, as part of these consortia, we can identify several elements or ingredients that are needed to make of them successful enterprises, yielding positive outcomes. For sure, the process takes a long time. It requires the presence of dedicated mentors and facilitators that can move effectively across countries, cultures, and languages. Language proficiency (both in English and other languages) is of utmost importance and is essential for day-to-day communication. Knowledge and respect for local cultures and a demeanor that demonstrates awareness on cultural nuances is essential. Highly relevant also is the actual benefit to local populations and the buy-in of local institutions and officials. Highest in the ranking, however, is the mentoring and training of local investigators, the promotion and funding of them as equals in the research enterprise.

In the case of the Colombia-U.S. and Argentina-U.S. collaborations that are the essence of chapters 4 and 5, it took decades to establish research sites, develop trust, build capacity, and succeed in getting and maintaining NIH grants that could be fully managed and implemented by competent local investigators working in the specific regions. The U.S.-based investigators provided ongoing mentoring, technical support, and expert advice, and they were available—either in person or virtually—to participate in the meetings of the investigators, particularly when key research decisions were made. These two large-scale research collaborations in Latin America have gone well beyond the "equity-attainment" and "task-shifting" strategies and have led to multiple and relevant publications in leading scientific journals, truly representing state-of-the-art research in the neurosciences.

Thus, despite the many problems and challenges, including the scarcity of specialty mental health professionals, the future of global mental health in Latin America appears much brighter than it did in the previous decade, thanks to the recent impetus of the field and the gradual appearance of agencies and philanthropists willing to support this important work.

Future directions for the field should include the following:

• Maintaining successful research and training collaborations, as well as forging new ones.
• Reinvigorating efforts to integrate mental health into primary care platforms, using successful models such as the one reported from Chile.
• Balancing the implementation of evidence-based approaches with new initiatives that emphasize "personalized medicine" and incorporate new developments in the neurosciences.
• Continuing to mentor and form new local investigators in all the regions of interest.
• Continuing to advocate for investments in this area by federal and private agencies.

ACKNOWLEDGMENTS

This book's editor and the authors of the various chapters appreciate the work, encouragement, and commitment of Rutgers University Press— Kimberly Guinta and Jasper Chang, in particular—in producing the current volume as part of a sustained effort to publish relevant works in the field of global health, a key priority at Rutgers University.

NOTES ON CONTRIBUTORS

MARIANA FIGUEREDO AGUIAR is an officer at the Fundación de Lucha contra los Trastornos Neurológicos y Psiquiátricos en Minorías in Buenos Aires (FULTRA), an agency that coordinates and supports research in Argentina.

CARRIE E. BEARDEN, PHD, is a professor and leading researcher from the Semel Neuroscience Research Institute at the University of California, Los Angeles (UCLA), who specializes in genetic studies of mental disorders. She is also a principal investigator for the NIMH project that focuses on the Paisa population of Colombia.

MARIA CALVO, MD, AND EDUARDO PADILLA, MD, are Argentinian psychiatrists who work in the mental health division of the region of Jujuy in northern Argentina.

GABRIEL DE ERAUSQUIN, MD, PHD, an Argentina-born psychiatrist, is professor and chair of neurology and psychiatry at the University of Texas, Rio Grande Valley. He has led research on the neurological and genetic aspects of schizophrenia in Kechwa populations in Argentina. He also has been mentored by Javier I. Escobar.

JAVIER I. ESCOBAR, MD, MSC, is an academic psychiatrist who is currently the dean for global health and a professor of psychiatry and family medicine at Rutgers–Robert Wood Johnson Medical School (RWJMS). An international expert on diagnosis and classification of mental disorders, he served on the task force that developed the fifth version of the *Diagnostic and Statistical Manual of Mental Disorders* (DSM-5) of the American Psychiatric Association, the most current classification system in North America. Escobar has been the principal investigator at Rutgers University for several NIH funded research projects in the past two decades. He has active ongoing collaborations in Spain as well as Latin America (Argentina and Colombia), and these serve as the main source for several of the chapters included in the book.

CARLOS LOPEZ JARAMILLO, MD, is professor and chair of psychiatry at the School of Medicine, Universidad de Antioquia, in Medellin, Colombia. Lopez

Jaramillo is an international expert on bipolar disorder and is one of the principal investigators of a large NIMH-funded project focusing on the Paisa population of Colombia. He has also been mentored for more than a decade by Javier I. Escobar.

HUMBERTO MARIN, MD, is a Colombia-born professor of psychiatry and practicing clinician also at Rutgers-RWJMS.

STANLEY NKEMJIKA, MD, MPH, is a Nigeria-born physician specializing in public health and a postdoctoral fellow in global health at Rutgers-RWJMS.

ETHAN PEARLSTEIN is a fourth-year medical student at Rutgers-RWJMS who has been very interested in the abuse of psychiatry in Spain and has been mentored by Javier I. Escobar for the past three years.

KATHLEEN J. POTTICK, PHD, a social psychologist and social worker, is a professor at Rutgers University and a member of the Institute for Health, Health Policy, and Aging Research at Rutgers–Biomedical and Health Sciences.

MIWA YASUI, PHD, is a clinical psychologist and an associate professor at the University of Chicago and the developer of the Culturally Infused Engagement model.

INDEX

Page numbers in *italics* represent figures and tables.

Printed in the United States
By Bookmasters